I'll Take Tomorrow

I'll Take Tomorrow

The Story of a Courageous Woman Who Dared to Subject Herself to a Medical Experiment —the First Successful Heart-Lung Transplant

MARY GOHLKE
with Max Jennings

M. EVANS AND COMPANY, INC.
NEW YORK

Library of Congress Cataloging in Publication Data

Gohlke, Mary.
  I'll take tomorrow.

  1. Gohlke, Mary. 2. Heart—Transplantation—Patients—United States—Biography. 3. Lungs—Transplantation—Patients—United States—Biography. I. Jennings, Max. II. Title.
RD598.G595 1985 362.1'97412 [B] 84-28803

ISBN 0-87131-458-4

M. Evans and Company, Inc.
216 East 49 Street
New York, New York 10017

Design by Diane Gedymin

Manufactured in the United States of America

9 8 7 6 5 4 3 2 1

To Dr. Bruce Reitz, who represents all the qualities which make man great and which take civilization a step forward, I dedicate this book.

Acknowledgments

I owe a deep debt of gratitude to many people. To Dr. Norman Shumway for his many years of pioneering work without which transplantation might still be a dream. To the nurses in the transplant program for their dedication to their profession and their caring. Without either I would not be alive to write this book. To Max Jennings, my friend and coauthor, without whom this book would never have been written, and to his wife Carol who supported both of us. To my many friends who sent me their love and encouragement daily.

Most of all to my husband Karl, my sons Chris and Luke, my mother and my family for their unceasing love and support which doesn't stop with the ending of this book. There are no adequate words to express my appreciation. All I can give is my loving thanks.

Authors' Note

This is a true story; however, some names have been changed.

FOREWORD

This is a fascinating and important story by one of today's medical champions. Mary Gohlke was the first patient to survive transplantation of the heart along with both lungs in an operation that was performed on March 9, 1981, at the Stanford University Medical Center. Whereas physicians and surgeons are often credited with courage and bravery, it is always the patient who deserves that credit.

In this chronicle we share the day-to-day fears, joys, and pains of a true pioneer, Mary Gohlke. The fact that she is alive and well following her historic operation makes it clear that her ordeal was worthwhile. As her story also makes clear, however, it is never a bed of roses for the patient who elects to undergo transplant surgery, whether it be a kidney transplant, heart transplant, or even heart-lung. There are fantastic problems related not only to the operation itself but also to its aftermath, the precise control of the immune system's reaction to the new organ. We in transplantation medicine tend to downplay the negative side of the various interventions that keep track of the body's immune response to foreign tissue. Mary Gohlke reminds us, however, just how difficult the nitty-gritty of living with a transplanted organ can be. The willingness of transplant patients to face and accept the enormous obstacles that follow any transplant procedure does bring us closer to the realization of what life is all about.

Although modern technology makes it possible to define death unequivocally, a suitable definition of what it is to be truly alive has yet to be found. This book by Mary Gohlke is a step in that direction.

Since Mary's surgery, twenty-three heart-lung transplants have been performed in twenty-two patients at the Stanford University Medical Center. Seventeen of those patients are alive and well. Numerous other centers throughout the world have joined Stanford in this approach to cardiopulmonary transplantation. As time goes by, we should expect the same good results from heart-lung transplantation that are now being achieved in so many institutions with heart transplantation alone.

All the doctors at Stanford, from Dr. Bruce Reitz, the surgeon-in-charge, to the newest intern, join me in saluting one of the genuine heroines of modern medicine, Mrs. Mary Gohlke.

NORMAN E. SHUMWAY, M.D., PH.D.
Professor and Chairman
Department of Cardiovascular Surgery
Stanford University School of Medicine

PROLOGUE

I FELT STRANGELY AT PEACE. I KNEW I SHOULD BE AFRAID. IN a few minutes, I would be given anesthetic and quietly go to sleep with a chance of never waking up. But I had lived too long with death as a constant companion to fear it now.

I looked around the operating room. It might be the last thing on earth I would ever see. Not a very romantic scene, the room bore little resemblance to those I had seen in the movies. My impression was one of clutter. Boxes, containing heaven knows what, were stacked along the white walls. A gleaming IV stand was near my right shoulder, and to my left was a maze of tubes and glass, the heart-lung machine that would soon sustain my life when my own failing heart and lungs were removed.

Behind me sat Dr. Mark Heilberman, the anesthesiologist, talking in quiet, gentle tones. He was explaining what everything was for and what was happening. Two nurses carefully laid out instruments for the operation. I could hear the soft murmur of their voices as they counted each item.

Bruce Reitz, whom I already thought of as a friend more than as a doctor, was pacing back and forth, impatient to begin. The sound of classical music was soft in the background. The work was vaguely familiar, but I couldn't remember the name. Bruce, like most surgeons, listened to music when he operated. Although his choice was classical, mine would have been jazz.

I knew that in the next room, two doctors, John Wallwork and John Pennock, were working to prepare the donor organs so the operation could begin. Wallwork, with his British accent and cheerful round face, had a smile that masked his deep compassion and dedication. Pennock, who seemed always to be hungry, had been there whenever I needed him most.

I looked back at Bruce Reitz, still pacing. I would see more of these three doctors in the next several weeks than would their families. They would keep me alive, I hoped. Many times in the coming weeks, they would not leave the hospital for days, mustering every bit of their skill and training and experience against the medical evidence that said Mary Gohlke had to die.

My part in getting to this point was over. The only thing I could do now was fight to live.

John Wallwork entered at last and spoke to Bruce. I couldn't hear the words, but I knew what he said. I began to tremble. The time had come. Dr. Heilberman started giving me the anesthetic. It had been a long, often hard, sometimes humorous journey to this operating room, but that was over now. What would be would be. Bruce Reitz had my life in his hands. I knew he would save my life. How could I be afraid?

ONE

IT LOOKED AS IF IT WAS GOING TO RAIN AGAIN. THE NORmally dry Salt River that bisects the Phoenix metropolitan area was already running in full flow, cutting the usually dry river crossings.

I would have to buck that traffic, and I felt frustrated and angry. I didn't want to go today; there was too much to do. I had already canceled one appointment with the cardiologist, and I was afraid to stand him up again. Besides, I had to find out what had happened to my normally inexhaustible energy supply. I looked into the mirror that morning and had to confess to myself I wasn't seeing the same old Mary. It was February, and I couldn't seem to bounce back from the pneumonia I had had in November.

I stood in front of the mirror over one of the twin sinks in the bathroom, putting on my makeup and sipping from a cup of coffee. Karl, my husband, was as usual shaving at the other sink. It was our morning routine.

"You going to the doctor today?" he asked. Karl had never been a nag. I knew how concerned he was.

"You could take the day off, honey," Karl said gently. "That place would not fall apart without you."

I just smiled, grateful, to that dear sweet man. "I'm going this morning, I promise." Karl was satisfied.

Lots of people called me a workaholic. It was true I was unable to get away from work for more than a few hours without missing it. But the truth was I was having the time of my life, and Karl shared that truth. I was advertising director for the *Mesa Tribune,* a lively daily newspaper in suburban Phoenix. It was the best job I had ever had, and I was determined to make the most of it.

And I was doing just that. I had a right to be proud of what I had accomplished. Advertising sales had doubled in the two years I had been on the job, and I was hell-bent on keeping up the momentum.

Drive and energy had carried me this far, but the energy had suddenly started to fade. I had seen several doctors; one tentatively suggested I was a victim of "executive burnout." It was one of many theories suggested by the doctors I visited. I finally decided to see a cardiologist for a treadmill test. Something definitely was wrong, and I was as confused as the doctors because the routine examinations showed no problems.

I put on my favorite blouse-and-pants outfit, reasoning that if the doctor wanted to examine my chest, it would be faster and easier to slip out of a blouse. I added a gold chain and earrings and brown ankle-strap shoes and checked myself in the mirror. I was vaguely troubled by the reflection. I looked tired. Bone weariness was in my eyes.

My eyes have always been the dominant feature of my face. My face is round and, like the rest of me, small, but my eyes are large and brown. It certainly was true in my case that the eyes are the mirror of the soul. Karl always said that anyone could tell how I felt, sick or well, angry or happy, by looking into my eyes. He also has always said they are prettiest when I'm happy. They sparkle. Today, the sparkle was gone. My eyes were dull and lifeless. I looked away from the mirror quickly. There was something in them I didn't want to see.

Christopher burst into the bedroom.

"Hey Dad, my car is messed up again," he began. "Can I have your car tonight?" At seventeen, Chris was a quiet, intense boy vaguely interested in school, but fascinated by automobiles.

Karl nodded permission, but I interjected, "I don't think you should go out tonight."

"Oh, Mom! You just worry too much," he said. He was gone before the discussion could be extended.

Karl finished dressing and was gone. I had only Lucas to get on his way before I could leave. At fourteen, all he needed was a kiss and a wish for a good day. I backed my Grand Prix out of the driveway and drove to work, my mind on what was ahead of me.

My route took me from the upper-middle-class area in the northern part of town down wide streets, laid out by Mormon pioneers in the early part of the century, to the heart of the city where the *Mesa Tribune* had been publishing practically since the city was founded. There was a slight nip in the February morning, but I found it refreshing. I love the winters in Mesa; it's the strength-sapping summer heat I could do without.

Two blocks from the paper, I slowed the car a bit to admire a giant lilac bush growing next to the street. It was covered with beautiful purple blossoms and would be that way for much of the winter. I was grateful for its beauty.

I parked in front of the paper in a spot normally left for customers because I would have to leave soon. Actually, I always have been terrible when it comes to parking. It's a family joke. I drive Karl crazy with my parking tickets. Once I found a policeman waiting for me when I returned to my car. He just had to see who had the audacity to park in a no-parking zone in front of a police station. The officer thought I was cute, but I got the ticket anyway.

I got a cup of coffee in the composing room and started to organize my day around the doctor's appointment. I waved to John Hanron, my sales manager, to follow me into my office. I knew I'd be gone most of the day and would have to explain to him what had to be done. We went over some sales fliers for a special issue.

"I've got too much damned work to do today," I complained to my secretary after John left. Pat Zeinbell frowned. She was determined.

"This is your second appointment with the doctor, and this time you're going to go even if I have to push you out the door," she said.

Although we had worked together only a few months, Pat and I had become close, and I knew that she, as much as anyone, knew something was wrong. I chain-smoked Pall Malls as we worked through the correspondence. As usual, I had no breakfast except for a cup of coffee.

Three and one-half hours later, I had worked my way through the snarled traffic across the Salt River bridge to the office of Dr. Mark Slater, a prominent Phoenix cardiologist. I had known Dr. Slater since he had examined me for an insurance policy I had bought while working for another publishing company a few years earlier. Dr. Slater, tall, with a touch of gray in his hair, was soft-spoken and attractive. I didn't know him well, but I trusted his competency.

I wanted to know why I had a sudden shortness of breath. I knew this was a symptom often associated with heart problems. And while I didn't like the idea of having this particular kind of test, I was convinced my previous examinations had failed to detect what it was that was wrong with me.

Dr. Slater's nurse took me in for an X ray. I waited several minutes in the examining room for the results, trying to read a copy of *The New Yorker,* but I couldn't seem to concentrate. The nurse finally came back and took me to another examining room for an electrocardiogram and a treadmill test.

The technician attached the tacky discs to my skin and had the wires hooked up in two or three minutes. When the results came out, the technician stared at the tape for a few minutes and mumbled something about doing the procedure again. She ran the test a second time, looked at the tape, and turned toward the door.

"I'll be back in a minute," she said. "Something seems to be wrong with the machine."

She was back in a moment with a new nurse who was very apologetic.

"Excuse me, Mrs. Gohlke," she said. "I'm going to take this one. The doctors were in here this morning fooling around with the equipment. Whenever they use the ECG they foul it up."

Her innocent-sounding remark alarmed me. The nurse was hiding something. I'd worked with people too long not to be sensitive to them. My co-workers kid me about my "gut feelings," but they respect them. They're usually right. This time I had the feeling there was nothing wrong with the machine.

The second nurse took the tape, left the room for a moment, and returned to tell me simply, "We're not going to do the treadmill test today." She left again, and in a moment Dr. Slater entered. He examined me carefully, concentrating mostly on the left side of my chest.

"I want you to come into my office," he said when he had finished. I dressed, irritated about not getting the treadmill test. That was the main reason I had come. I didn't have the time to be running back and forth. Anybody ought to be able to do the treadmill test, I thought. I thought that with the kind of treadmill I was on every day at work, this one had to be a snap.

Dr. Slater was seated behind his desk. He pointed to two X rays on display behind him.

"This is the X ray we did three years ago for your insurance examination," he said, pointing to the one on the left. "This is your heart then. It is normal, perfectly normal. The other one is the X ray we did today. Do you see this big dark spot?" He gestured dramatically to be certain I understood how big he meant. "That's your heart today."

I felt a twinge of alarm. My stomach was sending me signals. I pushed Slater. "Are you telling me I have heart trouble?"

"No," he said. "Not exactly. What I'm telling you is that you have a very serious disease called primary pulmonary hypertension. It really is a disease of the lungs. The blood vessels in your lungs close up. Your heart has to work harder all the time to pump the blood through them. As a result, it is enlarging due to overwork."

I wanted to scream at Slater, to urge him to get to the bottom line. But I did a good job of covering my feelings. He continued.

"Your heart has enlarged so much that every time it beats now it's hitting your rib cage. That's why you're so sore."

It was the first logical explanation I had had for the peculiar soreness in my chest that had bothered me for weeks.

"Okay," I said, trying to keep my voice steady. "Fine. What does all this mean?"

Dr. Slater looked at me steadily. "Primary pulmonary hypertension is a terminal disease."

I could scarcely breathe for a moment. I suddenly felt removed from that office. It was as if I saw myself from a distance sitting there as part of the scene. I am sure Dr. Slater could detect no reaction. I was numb inside and out.

Only one idea entered my mind. "How much time do I have?" Slater was evasive at first. I pressed him quickly because I wanted to know, and now.

"I don't like to make specific predictions," he said. "But I feel you have about five years."

For a few moments, I sat there, feeling nothing. I guess I didn't know what to feel. Then the anger began to build slowly but steadily until I was about to burst, as violent as I've ever been in my life. I sat staring at Dr. Slater's medical degrees, neatly framed and hanging on the wall. I wanted to smash them. He had no idea what was going on in my mind. Outwardly, I was calm. There was one more question I had to ask.

"What can you do for it?"

"Nothing really," he said. "I've only seen a few cases of it. There are a few drugs we can try, but there are no really effective vasodilators." I didn't even ask for an explanation of that term. My attention had stopped on the "nothing." After that, technical terms could have no meaning.

"You're telling me there's no pill or treatment I can take or anything you can do for me? You're telling me I have only five years to live?"

Dr. Slater grunted. I realized it was almost as difficult for the doctor as it was for me. He was a doctor, and he wanted to help me. He had worked for years to learn to save lives, and now he was helpless. Helplessness is a terrible feeling. We both knew that. My anger cooled as suddenly as it had come. Indeed, I wanted to comfort Dr. Slater, but my practical nature took over.

"I've got two kids to raise, and you're telling me I have five years to do it? What's next?"

"I'd like to have you in the hospital tomorrow to have a heart catheterization to confirm my diagnosis," Slater said. "It's the only sure way. I'd like to be wrong, but I'm 99 percent sure you have primary pulmonary hypertension. I'll make the arrangements to have you admitted."

I started to stand.

"Where are you going now?" he asked.

"To work," I answered. It had not occurred to me to do anything else.

"Why don't you go home?"

"For what? There's nobody home." My voice was hard, brittle. The anger was not gone. I turned and left.

It was a bright, warm day as I walked back to my car. The early morning chill had gone, replaced by the soft warmth that brings gladness to the Phoenix tourist bureau. The air was still and clear, and the sun, oblivious to my despair, seemed to radiate good cheer.

I was dying. It would take me an hour and a half to return across the river because of the traffic caused by the floods. I would have a long time to think.

I resolved nothing in that time. The anger returned in a slightly different form by the time I got to the office, though. "What the hell do I do now?" I thought. My mind was not working right, but I kept thinking, "How in the hell am I going to tell everybody?" The hardest person to deal with would be Karl. My hand strayed to the telephone, but I put it down without dialing. I couldn't tell him over the phone. I wanted him with me when I told him. Sometimes Karl worked late. I didn't want that today. I made a quick call to him, calming my voice.

"Was I right?" he asked. "Did the doctor tell you you've been working too hard?" I couldn't answer his question.

"We'll talk about it," I said. I repeated my question. "Can you come home early?"

"Sure," he answered. I knew from his tone he knew something was wrong, but he wouldn't press me.

For twenty minutes or so, I sat at my desk, aimlessly shuffling papers. Pat brought me a cup of coffee. I wanted to forestall any questions. Before she asked, I told her I was going into the hospital the next day.

"I have to have a test," was all I could bring myself to tell her.

My chief lieutenant, John Hanron, stuck his head in the door.

"Well, what did he have to say?"

"It was the shits," I responded. It was the best thing I could think of. Something in my voice told John he was dismissed. I hated to do it, but I felt lost. I couldn't sit there any longer. I left my office and walked down the hall to the office of Haney Womack, the general manager of the newspaper and my immediate boss. He was a man I had grown immensely fond of.

Haney and I must have made a curious sight when we walked through the plant together. He was six three, 230 pounds, and walked with a stride twice as long as mine. I'm five feet and weigh maybe 100 pounds if I'm carrying an encyclopedia.

I've always had to back away and look up at him to carry on a conversation. He called me "Shorty" and put more pressure on me than on anyone else who worked for him. I loved it. Haney knew how to get the most out of people, and he had pressured me into becoming the most productive ad director of his tenure. We had many battles, but we had respect for each other, and we developed an odd affection for each other.

Now, more than anyone in the building, Haney was the one I wanted to talk to.

The big man was seated at his desk going over computer reports of sales. It had never taken the two of us long to get to the point.

"I have to go into the hospital for two weeks," I began.

"What is it, Shorty?" Concern in his eyes betrayed the gruffness in his voice.

For the first time that day, I felt sorry for myself. My eyes filled, the tears running in a river down my cheeks. There was no easy way to tell Haney.

"The doctor told me I'm dying."

Haney's huge fist came crashing down on the desk.

"The hell you are!"

As always, when Haney was upset, his lips turned white. His eyes narrowed, and he looked at me carefully.

"Just what the hell have you got?"

"The doctor calls it primary pulmonary hypertension. It's sort of a corrosion of the blood vessels in the lungs. My heart is enlarged."

Haney was speechless.

"It's a rare disease," I said, rushing ahead with my explanation as if to reassure him. "He doesn't see it very often. He wants a heart catheterization to make sure, which is why I have to go into the hospital. The bottom line is this: I have about five years to live."

For the second time that day, someone told me to go home. Haney did it ever so gently. I was touched by the big Texan. Still, I refused. Deep down, I just couldn't face going alone to an empty house.

I went back to my office, calling John Hanron on the way. I first laid out carefully what he had to do during my two-week absence. Then I carefully told him about my condition. John is an ex-Marine with a thick Boston accent, a macho type in many respects, but with the kind of personality I like.

He wept openly. The two of us had worked together for a couple of years and had grown close. There was nothing for John to say. I felt sorry for him. He wanted to do something, but he was helpless.

I told my secretary, Pat Zeinbell, next. It began to get easier with her. I was amazed at how quickly I was adjusting to the task of telling people I was dying. It was remarkable that the human mind could accept something so incomprehensible so quickly and then immediately begin to adapt to the situation.

With Pat, I felt as if I were not really discussing anything that affected me directly; I might have been talking about a distant acquaintance. I suppose my mind was somehow allowing me to do what I had to do.

As I worked through the rest of the afternoon leading up to my conversation with Karl that night, I was astonished to realize I was subconsciously putting my life in order, setting priorities about how I would keep things together as my health deteriorated, how I would break the news to the kids. Again and again, I asked myself, How could I keep things together as I slowly died?

At 4 P.M., Dr. Slater called with my instructions for entering the hospital the next day. That was the last detail of a memorable "workday." The kids were home now so I decided to leave the office.

The children didn't sense anything was wrong. That was a relief to me. I was afraid they would see my face and start asking questions. Luke grumbled when I told him to clean up his room. As usual, it made a pigpen look clean and neat by comparison. I pulled steaks out of the freezer and started scrubbing potatoes to bake.

Chris washed his car, and Luke busied himself by carrying a seemingly endless supply of dirty glasses from his room.

They were so normal! Life was so good! I couldn't stand it. I went into the bedroom and sat down on the bed and cried. How was I going to tell the boys?

When Karl came home, we were in the family room watching television. His first question was about my day.

"The doctor said I have to go into the hospital tomorrow for a heart catheterization," I said. Karl's eyes narrowed suspiciously.

"What's the problem?"

"He says I have a disease, and the only way they can diagnose it properly is through catheterization.

Karl busied himself in the kitchen, peppering the steaks and firing questions at me.

I dodged the questions. "Let's wait until after dinner," I said. I didn't want to tell him with the children around. He nodded his acquiescence. He had always been a patient man; he would wait until I was ready to tell him.

Neither of us remembers much about dinner. After we finished, we went into the bedroom. I sat on a chair and Karl sat across from me on the bed. For the second time that day, I really let myself go. Karl came over and sat on the arm of the chair, holding his arm tightly around me until I could stop sobbing.

"I have a disease," I said, searching desperately for the right words. "It's called primary pulmonary hypertension. It's going to kill me. The doctor says I'm dying."

I could feel Karl's body grow rigid. Then his questions came rapidly.

"Dying? What does he mean, dying? How long do you have? How many years? Is there anything he can treat it with?"

After he allowed himself this bit of emotionalism, Karl, the scientist, started to analyze.

"Can this thing go into remission like cancer?"

I knew little more than he did, but I thought I could answer that. "It's a progressive disease, Karl. The doctor wasn't very encouraging about medication. They will try several things and see if they can do any good and if I can tolerate them. There is little chance of remission."

I was crying again. All my life I have been afraid to take medications because they almost invariably caused unpleasant side effects. I was growing frightened just thinking about it. I've always been the kind of person who could just read the label on a bottle of sleeping pills and go to sleep. It's one of the reasons I seldom drink anything stronger than coffee. Even one alcoholic drink has a big effect on me.

For some reason, the prospect of having to take a lot of medications suddenly took on huge importance, as if I could understand and fear that more than I could death itself.

For an hour, Karl and I talked quietly in the bedroom. I asked him repeatedly how we should tell the kids. We decided to wait until we had more information. And we simply didn't see any need to trouble them until we had to.

Taciturn by nature, Karl is used to approaching problems as an engineer. First he gathers facts. This was no different. It was as if he were unwilling to accept what I had said until he heard the facts firsthand and had analyzed them for himself. Even I did not know for sure what was going on in his mind.

He would tell me eventually, I knew, but first he had to come to grips with his own feelings. I knew he was that way, and I loved him.

The catheterization the next day was a grim

affirmation of Dr. Slater's diagnosis; the procedure was much worse than even my fertile imagination had conceived.

They strapped me in a device that looked like a canoe and secured my right leg so that it was absolutely immobile. The doctor made a small incision in my thigh and inserted the catheter, slowly working it up the artery while watching its progress on a televisionlike screen. The test clearly showed what Dr. Slater had diagnosed. My heart was greatly enlarged from trying to pump blood through the collapsing vessels of the lungs. The blood pressure in my lungs, of course, was abnormally high.

After the test, I felt well enough to have lunch, but I was plagued by persistent pain caused mostly by the incision in my thigh. Somehow, although I had thought I had made it clear that I was allergic to codeine, the message didn't get through to the hospital staff. A nurse gave me a painkiller, and I gratefully took it, unaware it contained codeine. Within minutes, I began to grow faint. By the time Karl had summoned help, I was in deep shock. The next two days were spent in intensive care.

When I was feeling somewhat better, Karl and I had more conversations with Dr. Slater, who confirmed his best guess that I had five years to live, a prediction that was to prove tragically optimistic. I had plenty of time to think as I rested over the next few days. I kept my attention on the practical matters. Dr. Slater had told me my diminishing strength would be better conserved if I did not work.

"But what will I do?" I asked. "I think working will help me cope with this better. I'm not a homemaker. More than that, I can't go home and wait to die. There's more to living than just keeping the body alive."

Slater seemed unimpressed by my speech.

"You're not going to be able to work the hours you've been working," he reminded me gently.

In those next few days, I would go over in my mind again and again how I would live out the time I had left. I vowed to keep my life and my home as normal as possible. Finally, I admitted to Slater what I said to no one, not even Karl.

"How am I going to function as a normal human being when I'm not normal? For chrissakes, face it, I'm not normal. I'm looking at a graveyard a few years down the road. I have a couple of kids who for five years are going to need me. Luke is only fourteen, and there isn't even a guarantee of five years."

It was a statement that needed no response. Although he didn't say so, Chris probably needed me more at that time than did the ebullient Luke, who was perpetually cheerful and busy. Chris, a junior in high school, so big, strong, and hardworking, seemed helpless in many ways. He was a strange mixture of boy and man. He was going to his first formal dance while I was in the hospital. How much more would I have to miss? I asked myself.

Two days before the dance, Chris visited me in the hospital and confided he had not yet rented his tuxedo. From my bed, I issued marching orders. Karl and Chris were sent out that day to the tuxedo rental department at Sears, and Chris was outfitted from head to toe. Luke took Polaroid pictures.

Chris, resplendent in his rented finery, showed up at the hospital to present himself for inspection. Seeing him standing there so strong and handsome, I was ecstatic. He looked terrific.

After he left, I wept in frustration. I should have been there to help him when he needed me. I cried softly almost until dawn, but now the grief was mixed with something else. The feeling in my stomach was not self-pity. I came to grips with it sometime that night. I was *afraid.* I knew I was going to die, and it was absolutely terrifying. What made that moment even worse was that I could not forget my fear even for a second, because each time my enlarged heart beat, it hit my rib cage. My chest was tender, and the beating of my heart hurt. It was like a clock saying, "You're dying, you're dying," each beat repeating the awful litany. It would be a long, long time before I could confide my terror to anyone, even my husband.

I learned something else that night, something only the terminally ill know. I learned the haunting loneliness. It's impossible to understand how alone a person can be until something like this happens. It's a loneliness that can't be helped by other people. There was no way I could articulate to Karl how I felt, so I didn't try. I was glad I could spare him that, at least.

TWO

MY WEEKLY VISITS TO THE DOCTOR WERE LIKE GETTING BAD report cards. Except there was nothing I could do to improve. I hated being helpless. I wanted to do something.

I had no reason to argue with Slater who with each visit told me the disease was progressing more rapidly than he had expected. I could feel it. It was as if I had something inside me, an intruder attacking from within. The intruder was growing stronger, and I was getting weaker.

The worst part was the realization that I was putting a terrible burden on Karl. There was nothing he could do to comfort me, and he knew it. Yet he never lost hope. The pragmatic scientist side of him yielded to blind hope in this area only.

I began working shorter hours at the paper simply because I ran out of gas every afternoon. I could not force myself to continue. I put more and more work on John Hanron, and he kept things running smoothly without complaining. My new secretary, Carole Doyle, was able to handle most of my correspondence without supervision, and that helped enormously. The efficiency of the two of them covered up my own diminished performance to a great degree. They were small rays of sunshine in the darkest part of my life.

Haney watched over me like a sheep dog, ready to pounce on anyone or anything that gave me any trouble. If he saw me after three in the afternoon, he'd almost physically throw me out. I knew the big Texan still couldn't accept the fact that I was dying. That was one thing we had in common. Neither could I.

One day he suggested I get the opinion of another doctor, a Texas doctor. I still don't know if he was kidding about the Texas part. I suspect not. Most Texans I know would be atheists if they didn't believe God was a Texan.

I talked with Karl about getting another opinion. Karl was instantly responsive. Together, we agreed we would find the best.

I had done a lot of reading about famed Houston heart surgeon Dr. Michael DeBakey. I relished the idea. Haney would love my choice because DeBakey was a true Texan.

From what I had read, DeBakey appeared to be my kind of person. He didn't listen to excuses; he just got the job done. I had heard he was hard on the doctors who worked for him. He didn't like failure. That struck a chord. He was a positive person.

The next day I called the Mesa Public Library and asked a librarian to look up DeBakey's address. In a few minutes, she had his phone number. I dialed and almost laughed out loud at the accent of his secretary.

"I want to come to Houston to see Dr. DeBakey," I said directly. I was put on hold a short time, then a man's voice came on the line. The accent, if anything, was even stronger, a nasal twang.

"How may I help you, my dear?" Dr. DeBakey asked. He listened while I quickly described my condition, ending with a single statement, "I want a consultation."

"Certainly," DeBakey said without hesitation. Then in a manner I would find typical, he inquired kindly about my travel arrangements and finances.

"Do you need help?" he asked gently.

"I'm okay," I answered. "I have insurance."

"Fine, I'll put you back on the phone with my secretary to make the arrangements," he said. "Have faith. We'll see what we can do to help you, my dear."

I will never forget his kindness at that moment. It certainly was what I needed.

Karl and Haney were delighted to hear I would make the Houston trip. Slater agreed I should have a second consultation, but he didn't offer any encouragement.

It was a beautiful warm day in early May when Karl drove me to the Phoenix airport. I love spring. Spring in the Valley doesn't have the sharp contrast with winter that I was used to in Buffalo. Yet the desert blooms in spring in Arizona, too, a reminder of life. Life was very precious to me. Both of us had hope. We were strangely happy driving to the airport. There was a possibility the legendary Dr. DeBakey might find a way to save my life. It wasn't a hope based on reason. DeBakey had promised nothing except to try. Ours was a blind hope springing, I suppose, out of fear and desperation.

I felt as if someone had put a warm, wet blanket over my head when I stepped off the plane in Houston. I took a cab to the hospital. By the time I arrived, I was exhausted and needed a wheelchair to get to the reception area.

There were about 150 people in the waiting room, and I was the only person in a wheelchair. I settled down for a long wait, but an orderly came up and asked me whom I was waiting to see. When I mentioned DeBakey's name, everything changed quickly. I was whisked to a small room where a clerk went over my insurance forms and admission papers. Then I was taken upstairs to a private hospital room. I started to feel like a celebrity of sorts because of the way I was being treated. It was nice thinking that just being a patient of DeBakey's generated this kind of treatment. It was a great tonic after the exhausting trip, and my spirits started to lift. I sat in the room for a few minutes just looking around, then changed into pajamas.

A nurse came in and found me sitting on the bed. She apologized.

"Why, honey, y'all have to sit on the bed and wait? Ah'm so sorry." Every word she spoke had at least two syllables. I warmed up to her immediately while she took my blood pressure and temperature and ordered my dinner.

Dinner, not to disappoint me, was a Texas-style welcome to the hospital—barbecued ribs with all the trimmings. It was delicious. I've been in many hospitals in my life, and most deserve the terrible reputation associated with hospital food. I've even heard rumors of patients who died in the afternoon just to avoid dinner. But not in Methodist Hospital. Every meal was a delight.

I soon learned that Dr. DeBakey wasn't in Houston and wouldn't arrive for three more days. He was in Egypt treating the recently deposed shah of Iran and wouldn't arrive until Wednesday. In the meantime, he had left instructions with his staff to begin the preliminary interviews and examinations with me.

His staff was very much aware I had arrived. After dinner, doctors trooped into my room in a steady stream to ask questions and take my medical history. They were frank with me. They had the chance to see only three or four cases a year of primary pulmonary hypertension, and they were curious.

I was kept busy the next three days having X rays taken and countless examinations. I was interviewed and re-interviewed by cardiologists and surgeons and other cardiovascular specialists. They were particularly interested in examining my enlarged heart, they said. Late Wednesday afternoon, a change came over the floor where I was staying. The air was laden with expectancy. Instantly, everyone seemed to be saying the same thing. DeBakey was back! I was incredulous at the great awe such a simple statement seemed to generate.

It was odd. Even today I can't explain it. It was as if God had come down from heaven. The news was circulated quietly, of course. DeBakey was at least one of the reasons Methodist Hospital was so quiet, in sharp contrast to the other hospitals I had known. The nurse explained this to me.

"He believes a person is supposed to be in a hospital to rest and not be bothered," she said. "God help anyone out in the hall making noise if he doesn't have to. Dr. DeBakey is real strict. There are a lot of sick people up here."

All I could say to that was "Amen."

An aide came in a bit later to inform me that I would see DeBakey later that evening. The orderly stopped just short of saying "the Great DeBakey," but that's clearly what he felt. Shortly after dinner, he returned with a wheelchair for my short trip to DeBakey's suite.

The waiting room was packed with all kinds of people, some on rolling beds, barely able to move, others sitting in rows of chairs. I stepped from my wheelchair and sat down next to a man who didn't speak to me. As I looked around, something about the room struck me as strange.

Then I realized what it was. *Everyone* in the room was holding the same book, even a man lying on a stretcher gasping for breath, obviously in the last stages of life. He had his arms folded over his chest, and he clasped a book. The name of the author was on the cover. It was Michael DeBakey.

I soon found where the books all came from. In the corner was a desk stacked high with volumes in three convenient sizes. There was a cheap paperback version of the DeBakey autobiography, a fancier paperback version, and the deluxe cloth version. The gasping man on the stretcher had opted for the expensive cloth edition.

I turned to the man next to me and asked bluntly, "Why the hell has *everybody* got those books?"

The patient, who turned out to be a physician from Florida who had had two previous bypass operations, assured me with a wink, "You'll see."

I settled down to wait and watch. As patients were called to the receptionist's desk, they were handed a piece of paper and asked to fill it out. When my turn came, I got my answers. The slip asked which version of the DeBakey book I wanted, if I wanted the doctor to autograph it, and if so, how I'd like the inscription to read.

In the case of the gasping man on the stretcher, a nurse came over, took the book from under his arms, and brought it back to the receptionist for him so that his order would be completed. It was explained to me that the books—paid for by the patient—would be autographed by DeBakey with the words requested and later delivered to our rooms. For the real fans, autographed pictures were available.

I was incredulous at first. Then I started to laugh. The world had tipped askew; everybody was nuts. But the physician sitting next to me didn't think it was funny. He had a deluxe copy of the book under his arm, ready for autographing. I still would like to know what he requested as his inscription. Later, I bought a book too.

By the time all the patients in the room had filled out their autograph slips and returned them with their books, the poor receptionist was surrounded by stacks of them and had to peer out from between the stacks. I sat in my chair and giggled like a schoolgirl. Dr. DeBakey was a great doctor, maybe, but the patients acted as if they were going in to meet Bob Hope. No doubt about it, this was show biz.

The other patients glowered at me as I giggled. I couldn't help it. It reminded me of when I was a kid and used to giggle in church and get into trouble. From time to time, with what I can only describe as a flourish, white-smocked doctors rushed into the waiting room and told a patient breathlessly, "*The* doctor will see you now."

I felt as if I were waiting to see a great holy man who would simply lay his hands on my head and heal me. The comparison was inescapable. I giggled again.

At last my turn came. I was ushered into a tiny cubicle and sat in my robe and pajamas for a few minutes, still chuckling to myself.

The door popped open and there stood this little bitty old man. After the buildup, I had expected Dr. DeBakey to be as tall as an oak tree and twice as strong. He was dressed in a green surgical uniform, as if he were prepared to spring into the operating room at any moment. He was followed by three doctors who kept as close to him as they could. They all tried to jam into the tiny room where I sat. I presumed the doctor closest to Dr. DeBakey was in the greatest favor and that there was some kind of pecking order implied by their positions in line. The doctors all had their arms folded as if they were about to operate and couldn't touch anything. Dr. DeBakey seemed oblivious to the appearance created by his retinue or by the scene in his waiting room, which could have been created by the writers of M.A.S.H.

"Hello, Mary, I'm Dr. DeBakey," the little man said. "How are you feeling?"

"Just fair," I said simply. I *was* glad to be examined by this man. His presence was comforting.

"I have gone over all your records," DeBakey said. As he began to discuss my case, I could tell that he had, indeed, prepared himself well before talking with me. From his study of the heart catheterization, DeBakey said he could tell me unequivocally that I had primary pulmonary hypertension; there could be no other diagnosis. He told me, as Dr. Slater had, that there was no cure, but he said he wanted to try a few medications to see if they would improve my condition.

Then, unexpectedly, he blurted out, "I understand you have a couple of moles."

"Moles?" I repeated, surprised. Here I was, dying, talking to the great Dr. Michael DeBakey, and he wanted to look at moles. Who gives a damn about moles at a time like this, I thought. Apparently, members of DeBakey's staff who had examined me earlier mentioned the moles in their reports, one on my ankle and the other on the outside of my left thigh.

Dr. DeBakey pulled up the leg of my pajamas and stared intently at the mole on my ankle and at the other one on the outside of my thigh. He told one of his aides he wanted a dermatologist the next day to remove the mole on my ankle.

"I don't like the looks of it," he said, without explaining further. I let the matter pass. It was one of the few times I didn't press a doctor for an explanation of something I didn't understand. But the mole on my ankle just didn't seem important to me.

DeBakey listened to my lungs for a few minutes. As he worked, I watched his face. I found myself strangely reassured, comforted.

"We are going to try some different medications," he repeated. "I don't want you to worry. You never know in these matters what is going to happen, but your doctor was right in the diagnosis. You have a very rare disease, and there's not a whole lot we can do for it at this time."

Then he held out the tiniest hope. He told me he could tell patients they would die, and then he would see them again years later because no one could be certain. There is more to the human condition than simple technical analysis, he said.

"I'll see you again," DeBakey said, already turning to rush away, followed in quick step by the tall blond doctor and the two shorter ones. I speculated that if DeBakey were to stop too quickly, the aides would stumble into one another and the whole column would collapse like a string of dominoes.

Back in my room, I replayed in my mind the waiting room scene and Dr. DeBakey's hilarious entry into my cubicle, followed by his obsequious attendants. I laughed out loud and called Karl to describe it all to him before I forgot. I was still laughing when I got him on the phone, and soon he joined in. We both forgot everything else but the humor of that moment. It was the first laugh we had had in months.

Before I went to bed, I was examined by still another doctor. I realized that, everything else aside, Dr. DeBakey was concerned about me. He wanted to help and would spare no resources. If another doctor might have an idea, he was willing to try it. I was grateful for DeBakey's sincere care. It was indicated to me in ways I didn't quite understand: his manner, his knowledge of my records, his attention to what I considered minor things. He even worried about that damned mole. I felt his presence. I believed in him, and I believed that he was sincere in telling me I had to believe in myself. I, too, felt I had been in the presence of a great man.

There were a million stories about DeBakey circulating around the hospital. For example, a nurse told me about the time Dr. DeBakey was visiting a friend a few hundred miles from Houston. He spotted a man coming down the street whose face showed signs, long familiar to DeBakey, of oxygen deprivation. In an instant, DeBakey made his diagnosis. He was looking at a man with heart trouble.

On the spot, he took his bag out of his car, asked the stranger if he would step into his friend's living room, and performed an examination. The startled patient was thought by everyone in the small town to be retarded, but DeBakey knew the mental problems were caused by lack of oxygen to the brain. The blue-faced man was dirt poor, but Dr. DeBakey paid for the man to come to Houston and have the operation that eventually gave him a normal life.

I went home the following Sunday, uplifted for some reason by the Houston journey, and plunged again into work. I had learned at Houston that I slept better if I took a little oxygen at bedtime. I had oxygen delivered the next Monday to my house. I started sleeping better, and some of my energy returned.

For a few days, I was almost my old self, moving like a whirlwind, getting things done with a gusto I hadn't known in months. I was enjoying myself, but in the back of my mind I knew it couldn't continue. In a few weeks, I began to grow weary again. I never was in pain, but the weariness began coming earlier and earlier in the day. It was overwhelming, very hard to describe. It was a bone weariness. Sometimes it would take me five minutes just to push back from my desk and summon the energy to stand up. I felt as if I had run a race and couldn't catch my breath.

I began going home again in the middle of the afternoon and lying on the bed, gasping oxygen from the tanks that had become a permanent fixture in the bedroom. My assistant, John Hanron, gradually took on more and more responsibility. Now, the late night phone calls on production problems I used to take were routinely being routed to John. Still, I struggled on, insisting on getting up at 6 A.M. every day, visiting with Karl, and then going to the office. Karl and I have always had our best talks in the early morning, and I wasn't going to give up this part of my life.

The weekly visits to the doctor were slow mental torture. The news always was bad. Dr. Slater was astonished at how rapidly the disease was progressing. I was warned repeatedly that my reservoir of strength was limited and that the energy expended at work would take away from what I had left to spend with my family. This troubled me. I felt guilty and talked to Karl about it. He was understanding, but he pressed me.

"Honey, quit. We can manage without your working," he said. "You are a helluva a lot more important to me than a few bucks."

Finally, I admitted to Karl that the reason I could not quit work was that I was afraid to. I was beginning to fear being alone, and I hated coming home in the afternoons to an empty house. Fear began to haunt me, and I found it difficult to talk about it to anyone.

One morning in late June, I was getting dressed in the

bathroom and Karl was shaving at his sink. I was putting on makeup, staring at my reflection in the mirror. Suddenly, I froze.

It was the eyes, my eyes. They were dull, dead. The sparkle was gone. My eyes always had been my prettiest feature, but there was no denying the truth now.

"Karl, come over here," I said. My voice was unsteady.

Puzzled, he quit shaving and walked over to my side.

"My eyes. Look at my eyes. Karl, I'm dying."

He put his arms around me, but he didn't deny anything. That would have been useless. There was nothing for him to do or say. I sat on the edge of the bed with his arms around me and wept. Karl was dry eyed but granite-jawed. There was absolutely nothing more he could do for me. It was the loneliest moment of my life. I had the haunting realization that you can share anything in life with others, but in the end, you die alone.

THREE

On November 3, 1935, Bernadine Carmina, née Wilson, gave birth to a seven-pound, two-ounce baby girl. The child was named after Bernadine's mother, Mary. I was that child.

My first memories are of the lively, crowded home of my grandparents. It was noisy and filled with love because there were always so many there. My mother had been married at seventeen to a handsome, hardworking Sicilian, Joe Carmina. The marriage didn't work. It probably would be better to say it didn't even come close to working, and my parents separated when I was only a few months old.

The neighborhood where my grandparents lived was in the predominantly Irish Catholic south side of Buffalo, New York. Mary and "Butch" Wilson raised eleven children including my mother in the two-story row house that was my first home. The houses were all alike—worn and weatherbeaten on the outside, clean and warm within. Each had a tiny backyard. Ours was dominated by a huge tree. I learned to climb almost as soon as I could walk.

The people I don't remember as well as the tree. I remember they all worked hard all the time, and they lived hard. I guess that neighborhood could be called a ghetto, but nobody told us we didn't have enough, so we were happy.

My mother worked in a department store to support the two of us. She had worked since she was sixteen. In a family of thirteen, everyone works. When I was nine, Mother opened a restaurant, doing all the cooking herself and tending the bar. Sometimes she was so tired she slept on a cot in the back instead of coming home. Most of the time during those years I spent with my grandmother.

My mother married again to a kind, divorced man whose son, Bill, was younger than I was. I loved my little brother, and I protected him fiercely. I still would, I guess, if he needed me.

We lived about two blocks from my grandparents' home, and I continued to spend most of my time there. It was a very happy place, always spotless and fragrant with the smell of fresh-baked bread. The neighborhood was a rowdy, noisy place which demanded that you spoke up if you wanted to be heard. I learned early to be heard, especially when company dropped by, which was often. There was always room for one more. My aunts ranged from three to twenty years older than I and were known in the neighborhood as the "Beautiful Wilson Girls." A steady stream of suitors came by.

My voice and spirit grew faster than my body. I was a tiny little tomboy who loved playing hockey and football with the boys. One year my playmates bought me a set of pads. I often drove my grandmother to the brink of despair when I came home, dirty, my dress torn from playing football or fighting.

"Girls shouldn't be fighting," she'd chide me gently as she patched up my wounds. I would be silent. I didn't agree, but in my home you didn't talk back to your elders. In my neighborhood you had to stand up for yourself or fall by the wayside. There was no middle ground.

My early education was in the hands of the Sisters of

Mercy at St. Monica's parochial school. In my opinion, they were poorly named. The children were too poor to wear uniforms, but in every other way, the traditional discipline was in place. I was unsuited to accept the nuns' teachings almost from the beginning. I couldn't accept things on faith. I wanted to know why and how. I loved my religion and wanted to know more. I was particularly aggressive in my questions about religion.

"How could someone who was a virgin have a baby?" I asked again and again without getting an answer that satisfied me. Where I grew up, everyone knew where babies came from at an early age.

"How could the pope be Christ on earth?" The sisters didn't like that phrasing. "Why is it a sin to feel pride when you do your job well?" I was a good student. I worked hard, and I was uncomfortable with the notion that it was wrong to feel proud of what I had done.

I escaped by reading—poetry, fairy tales. I read all the books about the lives of the Catholic saints. I liked and admired some, but I thought some of them were dull. Especially those who hurt themselves. The nuns didn't appreciate my opinion. Sometimes I think I made them uncomfortable.

I got into trouble several times by refusing to go to confession. I felt I had nothing to confess. How many sins can a ten-year-old commit? From the nuns I learned that Christ had said, "Bless the little children," but I saw little blessing from the sisters. I solved the problem by making up sins to confess. I told the priest that I talked back to my grandmother, something I never did; it was unheard of in our family. I told him I lied; I hated lying. I confessed that I didn't do my work in school. I was an exemplary student, except for my unacceptable questions and my flat-out refusal to accept the teaching that it was wrong to have pride. I felt guilty about lying to the priest, but I figured God would understand. When the sisters could stand no more of my sharp tongue, I was ordered to go before the pastor, Father Fitzhenry. I was terrified. I would be doomed to hell. My mother would kill me.

Father Fitzhenry, who was my grandmother's age, was famous for his temper and his false teeth. When he was angry, he clicked his teeth. When I told him why I had been sent, he became angry with me and his teeth clicked. I was terrified I would giggle. The good father easily worked out a suitable punishment. I had to go to the grocery on the corner and buy a six-pack of Simon's beer and take it to the pastor—every day—as penance for my sins. I had to leave school for a short time to do it. I felt a little guilty because I liked my penance.

I used to sneak into the boys' club to shoot pool and play basketball. Several times I was caught and was escorted out with the admonition "You should be learning to sew." I didn't want to learn how to sew; shooting pool was more fun.

It was about this time at St. Monica's that I realized I liked to sing. I had a good voice and I was soon singing solos in the Mass. I loved it. My taste wasn't restricted to religious music. I saw every musical made in the forties, often sitting through a movie two or three times. I scraped up the money to buy "Hit Parade" songbooks so I could learn the words to the latest hits.

Our parish was too poor to have a music department, but once a week a nun came to school to teach voice and music. She was the most beautiful creature I had ever seen in my life. She had the face and voice of an angel. I loved her, I adored her. She was crippled and wore a huge shoe because one leg was shorter than the other.

Sister Marcia, the principal, found out about my new love and it gave her a new weapon. In Sister Marcia's view, I was making poor progress in religion, and she was particularly upset by my pride, which she viewed as evil. More than anything else, Sister Marcia reasoned, I would hate to miss my singing lessons. She was right. It broke my heart when, as a punishment, I was forbidden to go to music class and instead was sent to sit alone in another room to wait out the time. The tactic worked in one sense. I became a model student toward the end of the fifth grade, but that injury at the hands of Sister Marcia was the first of many that would someday drive me from the Catholic church.

When I graduated from eighth grade, I was not much bigger than I had been in the fifth grade. Although my body just wouldn't seem to grow, my will certainly had. Mother wanted me to go to Mount Mercy Academy, but by this time I hated the Mercy nuns. I wanted to go to Mount St. Mary's, which was on the other side of town. I knew that the Sisters of St. Mary was a good teaching order and the nuns would not be the harsh disciplinarians I found the Mercy Sisters to be. Mother, rather than send me there, ordered me to South Park High, heartbroken that I refused to go to Mount Mercy.

I enrolled in public high school, but I didn't want to go there. I promptly started skipping classes. When the truant officer caught me and dragged me in front of my mother, I told her the truth. My stepfather, who was not a Roman Catholic, intervened for the first time with Mother's handling of me. He told me he would arrange my enrollment in Mount St. Mary's, and he did.

I didn't do well, mostly because I had missed so many days, which put me far behind my classmates. Then my appendix ruptured, and I was in bed for thirty days. The nuns urged me to start my freshman year over. Instead, I decided I'd had enough of school. I would educate myself. I found a new place to go. I abandoned the boys' club for the local library. The librarian and I struck up a friendship based on my frequent visits. I began to devour anything that struck my fancy: history, literature, biographies of all types. I was still in school, I was fourteen, and the sisters tried to help, but they were too late. I was plagued by guilt because I simply could not accept intellectually the teachings of the Catholic church.

I dropped to part-time status in school when I got my

first job: folding sheets in a laundry. I had to fold a certain number in a day, and I was paid by the piece. My supervisor soon realized I was too small to fold sheets properly, so I was assigned to folding towels. The job lasted only two weeks before the laundry workers went on strike. I learned plenty from the tough crude women who devoted themselves to survival in that south Buffalo neighborhood. I learned that survival is your own responsibility. I felt, rather than learned, that there must be more to life than this.

I found another job in what I remember as a bag factory. It was a company that made pillow cases out of empty grain sacks. My job was to fit the bags to a large machine that blew the grain dust off the sacks and to fold them. I lasted two days. They were afraid the suction of the machine would suck me in instead of the dust.

By the time I was seventeen, I had my first selling job—in the costume jewelry department of Adam, Meldrum and Anderson's department store. For the first time in my life, I came into regular contact with people who had a different, more pleasant life-style than I did. I didn't envy them, but became determined to change my own.

I soon was obsessed with the idea of moving away from my home after my mother married for the third time. My new stepfather, Bill Martin, was very good to me, but I was determined to stay in my neighborhood no longer. I knew there was nothing there for me. If I stayed, I would become like a lot of my girlfriends who got married and had three or four kids and a husband who bounced them off the walls. It was a rough, rough area. I was maturing now and was no longer protected by the relative tranquillity of my grandparents' home. In that Irish-Catholic enclave, people worked hard, drank hard, and lived hard.

To this day I credit my grandmother for keeping things in perspective for me. In the squalor of what was an industrial slum, the Wilson home was a shining example of something better. Every day, Mrs. Wilson washed from her windows the grime poured out by a nearby chemical plant and presided over a household where order prevailed. My grandmother was no philosopher, but she taught me something many philosophers miss: you are not responsible for where or how your life starts, and you can't help what fate hands you, but you are responsible for what you do with your life.

One evening, my parents got into a loud argument and my mind was made up for me. I packed a small bag and announced that I couldn't stand to hear them fight anymore. I left and never returned.

FOUR

I HAD SET OUT ON A NEW COURSE AND WASN'T ABOUT TO waver or turn back. My new life, I resolved, would be better than the one I had left. I possessed little but a fierce determination and a knowledge of survival gleaned from the streets of south Buffalo.

Being on my own was exciting at first. I moved to the section of north Buffalo known as the university area, so named because it was then the home of the University of Buffalo. I rented a room and got a job.

The room cost me $10 a week with a bath down the hall I shared with several other roomers. I paid my rent, in cash, at the beginning of each week.

My first job on my own was waitressing at a Colonial House restaurant directly across the street from the university. I was only seventeen, but I had worked lunchtime and after school at my mother's restaurant since I was nine and so had more experience than most of my co-workers. I soon advanced to night manager.

The initial excitement of being on my own wore off quickly, replaced by a feeling of loneliness. I visited my parents and grandparents on my days off, but the rest of the time I was alone. I had left most of my old friends behind. I spent my days at the library, losing my loneliness between the covers of a book.

The clientele of the restaurant was predominantly college students, and I soon began to make friends. One man—I thought of him as an older man, but you don't have to be very old to gain that title from a seventeen-year-old—used to come in late at night when business was slow. He usually wore gray work clothes, and I knew he worked at the university. I thought he might be a janitor or workman. We'd often talk, and I found him an interesting conversationalist on almost any subject. He was a simple, warm, friendly man. I eventually learned he was the head of the department of physics at the university. It was many years later that I learned he also proofread encyclopedias. This professor was the first real intellectual I had ever come to know well, and from him I gained a good deal of knowledge, knowledge about people more than anything else.

A few months into my new life I met a boy I liked in particular. He was tall and skinny, and best of all, he was totally unlike most of the boys in the neighborhood where I was raised. Instead of being a loud, tough brawler, Bob was paying his way through college as a professional musician. He played the accordion (which I hated) and the trumpet, and he was studying psychology.

I began spending more time with the students on campus. We spent endless hours in discussions about anything that came up, but always with an eye to making the world a better place. Like most college students, we could solve the world's problems by 4 A.M. I began to attend classes without paying for them. It was easy to wander into the large lecture classes and take a seat in the back. I did this for two years, usually choosing anthropology or sociology.

Not all my friends were associated with the university. I became friends with Rena, who owned a small restaurant below the room where I lived. Sometimes, during the day, when Rena was very busy, I would volunteer my help for a few minutes. It was natural; she needed help, I knew how, I gave it. Finally I took a job at the smaller restaurant for more money, and soon I knew everyone on the block.

Next door to Rena's restaurant was a florist shop run by Kathleen and Danny Madden. They often stopped in Rena's for coffee or a sandwich. We soon became friends. Kathleen and Danny were the most cultured people I had known. Kathleen dressed stylishly and catered to a wealthy clientele.

It was not long before I was working at the florist shop where I first learned of my ability to sell. I knew little of flowers and was unable to identify most of them. I was learning about people, however; and the first plant I learned to name was the azalea. Thereafter it made little difference what kind of a plant you came into the shop to purchase, you left the shop happy with your azalea. The Maddens' supplier of azaleas wondered about the sudden rush on the plants, but he never complained. I was soon making funeral baskets, watering plants in the greenhouse, and turning out bridal bouquets. I grew to love Kathleen and Danny, who in turn fell in love with the tiny energetic little girl they had hired. I began to regard them as second parents.

I continued to take my coffee breaks at Rena's restaurant and often ate dinner there. I began to talk to one of the customers, a quiet, intense engineering student named Karl Gohlke. Karl often ate alone, working the daily crossword puzzle in ink while he ate. I was fascinated by this man. He was different from most of the students I knew, a little older, a little quieter, and I thought at first, a little aloof. As I came to know him better, I learned that the seeming aloofness was a mask for his shyness. Rena could see more than I could at nineteen. She told me, "Never mind those other guys you go out with, there's the one for you."

Another way in which Karl was unlike the other students I knew was that he only attended college at night. He worked full time days at Bell Aircraft. Still, he was carrying nearly as many credit hours as most of the full-time students I knew. I was fascinated and a little frightened by him. He was the most intellectual person I had ever known. He seemed to know something about almost any topic.

We had many conversations in the restaurant before Karl finally asked me out. He liked to drive, and on our first date he took me for a drive in the country. We talked animatedly until I suddenly realized it was 11 o'clock and I was on a rural road with a man I really didn't know that well.

"Take me home," I ordered suddenly, and Karl, embarrassed, turned the car around and drove me home in near silence. But he wasn't angry.

After that, Karl began to drop by the flower shop or we would eat dinner together at the restaurant nearly every day. I began to see the warm gentle man behind the intellectual facade. Our conversations quickly became more personal. We talked of our ideas, our hopes and dreams, our families, and the problems of our love life. We were falling in love. One night we were out driving and Karl stopped the car, turned to me, and said, "Mary, you have to marry me." That was it, no proposal, no choice—I didn't want one.

We had a traditional wedding, at least by the Gohlke family standards. It was in the Methodist church in Alexander, New York. It made no difference to me what kind of church I was married in. I had the man I wanted.

Karl's career as an engineer at Bell Aircraft flourished. He was working on a secret project related to missile guidance systems. I was never sure what he was doing. Karl was very closemouthed about his work. He was very good at it, a fact I learned from some of our friends who worked with him. A few months after our marriage, Bell transferred Karl to Oxnard, California, where he was assigned as a civilian engineer to a project at the nearby Point Mugu

Naval Base. I was twenty years old when we moved. It was the first time I had lived outside Buffalo. We drove across the country, the first time I had ever done anything like that. Karl had traveled quite a bit before we met, but every new sight was a delight to me and he shared my joy. On the way to California, we stopped at the Grand Canyon. The early morning sun was reaching into the canyon when we first saw it. The canyon was so deep and created such an overwhelming sight of towering rock and vastness that I couldn't speak for a moment. Then I whispered to Karl, "Now there is God." Karl put his arms around me. He knew what I meant.

We were deliriously happy in California. We made friends. We traveled on weekends, seeing most of southern California. I was disappointed when the job was done and Karl was reassigned back to Buffalo. We had a month off and took a leisurely trip across the country. We stopped in Idaho to visit friends of Karl's from his navy days. Then we visited Yellowstone National Park; I fell in love with the bears.

When we returned to Buffalo, we rented an apartment and bought the first furniture I had ever owned, a Danish modern living room set. I worked for an insurance company and in the book department of a department store. We entertained friends often and started saving to buy a home. We began to talk about having children. Many of our friends were college educated, engineers like Karl, and virtually everyone had at least completed high school. I should have been the dummy in this crowd, but I found I had no trouble entering into their conversation. But I nurtured a secret guilt. I had never told Karl I had not completed high school. In fact, when we first met, I had told him I had graduated from high school. One night I finally confessed and told Karl I wanted to finish school. He was stunned.

"Why you damned fool," he said. "You could have been going to school all this time. Don't be ashamed, Mary.

If you want to go to school, go. Don't be ashamed of what you didn't do—change it."

Nearly one year later, when I had finally struggled through the mysteries of algebra, much to Karl's amusement and despair, I earned my high school diploma. It was a proud day.

Then Karl got word that he would be assigned temporarily to a military project in Fort Huachuca, an isolated military post in southern Arizona, not far from the Mexican border. I was excited. I remembered the happy times in California. But it turned out to be nearly the worst five months of our marriage. We lived in a trailer park about five miles from Sierra Vista. We and two other families—the Roselers and the Alabrans, who worked for Karl and had come with us from Buffalo—nearly doubled the population of the trailer park. The most exciting pastime I could devise was that of watching the gophers scamper around the trailer. There was even a minidrama in this because the trailer park's owner was trying to kill the gophers, who were destroying the few scrawny trees he was attempting to grow. I was definitely on the side of the gophers. The only other amusement was reading. The librarian at the military base couldn't believe that I actually read all the books I checked out.

Leaving Fort Huachuca was like getting out of prison. As we drove through Phoenix on the way back to Buffalo, Karl said suddenly, "We're going to live here someday." I didn't answer. I was sure the heat was affecting his mind.

When we returned to Buffalo, we were still talking about having a family. But I became ill. My ovaries were loaded with fibroid tumors and I would have to have a hysterectomy. Fortunately the tumors were benign. The surgeon removed fifteen tumors and, with the operation, my ability to bear children. It hurt, not the physical pain, but I lost part of what I was.

Karl and I applied to county officials to adopt a baby. After months of meetings and consultations, I was disgusted and discouraged. The counselor at the adoption agency was a million years behind the times. She still believed in "bad seed" and was trying to line up a baby worthy of us. I told her what a baby "worthy of us" was: one that I could hold and love. My opinion wasn't appreciated. She reminded me of the Mercy nuns.

I talked to my doctor about a private adoption. He said it would take time. We bought our first home that summer, and I entered college at the University of Buffalo in the fall of 1963. Less than six weeks later, in October, I received the call I'd been waiting for.

"Hello, Momma," my doctor began. My knees grew weak as I listened. "You're the mother of a bouncing baby boy." It's been over twenty years since that day, but five minutes after our conversation I couldn't have described it in more detail. I had heard all I wanted to hear.

I wanted to call Karl at work, but I was afraid he would get so excited that he would have a wreck on the way home. I waited an eternity until he got home, and we drove immediately to the hospital that night to see our firstborn—Christopher Michael.

FIVE

IT WAS A HAPPY TIME. I QUIT SCHOOL WHEN CHRIS WAS BORN and enjoyed the role of wife and mother. Three years later a second child entered our life and my heart. We brought Lucas home from the hospital when he was four days old. Again the adoption came through the help of my doctor.

The years rushed by and soon both boys were in school. When Luke started school, I was filled with a mixture of joy and sadness. The boys were growing up. I loved watching and helping them grow, but I would never again hold them to my breast as I fed them. I knew there was still much to do in raising them, that they would need me for many years still. But their infancy was over, and henceforth I would spend much of the daytime alone.

I went back to work selling advertising space for a telephone directory. It was the first really good job I ever had. I enjoyed the advertising field and found sales a welcome challenge. The extra income helped and we were very comfortable. There was trouble brewing, but I couldn't, or wouldn't, see where it was leading. An undercurrent of tension was building between Karl and me. We no longer talked to each other as we used to.

Nearly every vacation we went West. Karl had always

loved the West. One evening in the late winter of 1974 Karl told me he wanted to quit his job and move West. The company he worked for was stagnating and so was he. He called an old friend in Scottsdale, Arizona. We flew out to Arizona for a few days, and when Motorola offered Karl a job, he decided to accept.

I had never particularly cared for the desert. I dislike the heat and the compression of the seasons. Cactus is not my idea of a plant. Still, I was willing to go, even though it meant I had to quit my job. I could sympathize with the way Karl felt about his. Stagnation is like a slow death. Maybe the move and a fresh start for him would repair the small tears in the fabric of our marriage.

We sold our home and moved. I was shocked at the cost of real estate in Arizona. Our new home cost half again as much as the one we sold in Buffalo and wasn't nearly as nice. The boys entered school and I found work with a publisher of television directories. The opportunity was excellent: I'd be an officer of the corporation, the only drawback being that I had to travel often. My selling trips frequently took me to nearby states, and I would be gone for a few days. The company was just starting out, and Karl and I put our remaining money into it. I put my time into it, often working fifteen or sixteen hours a day. A year later I began to suspect some of the dealings in the company were not as they should have been. I'd been so involved in selling, in bringing in the revenues, that I'd paid scant attention to the finances. I guess I was still a little naive. I trusted our president when he said the company was doing fine. I only knew I was bringing money in.

One day the bank called me. Our notes were overdue and they couldn't get a satisfactory explanation. I immediately began to check with our other creditors. I heard the same story everywhere: our payments were behind and our checks were bouncing all over the Phoenix valley. I and the other officer of the corporation confronted the president. He tried to stall us and wouldn't show us the books. We sought legal help, and on our lawyers' advice we returned all of our stock and resigned from the corporation.

I had nothing to show for my year of toil. I had put my best efforts, our savings, my hope into that business and it was gone. With it went my marriage. Karl and I stayed together for a few months longer, but we were no longer a pair. It wasn't because of the business failure. It wasn't Karl's fault and it wasn't mine. We had been growing apart even before we had left Buffalo. Trying to pinpoint reasons didn't help. 1977 dawned to find our marriage over.

I moved into an apartment. The boys stayed with Karl at first. I was lonelier than I had ever been in my life. At night I would cry myself to sleep. I found another job in advertising sales. The days were better than the nights. At least I was busy then. I went back to working fourteen-hour days. The best time of the day was when I called the boys. I went over to see them often, and I'd take them with me on weekends. Once I decided to introduce the children to a man I had started to date. They were cold and rude. I could see they were hurt. I didn't try that again.

I worked for Charles Wahlheim, a charismatic, impulsive man who had been one of the key executives in a major newspaper chain by the time he was in his mid-thirties. Now, he was trying to make a go of a free distribution weekly in Phoenix. In 1978 Cox Enterprises, an Atlanta-based newspaper chain, bought the *Mesa Tribune,* a small suburban daily. Wahlheim became publisher. He offered me a position in the advertising department. A few months later I took it.

Karl had bought a town house in Tempe, only a few miles from the *Mesa Tribune.* He offered me the town house. I had seen Karl often since we were divorced, usually for a few minutes when I picked up the boys. But sometimes I'd stop in for a longer talk. We were never bitter toward each other, and when I had a problem, business or personal, I'd talk it over with him and sometimes ask for his advice. I always valued his opinion. He still balanced my checkbook.

When he offered me the town house, I grabbed it. I'd have my children with me again. I felt a crushing guilt about leaving them. I knew Karl would care for them, love them, and raise them well, but these facts meant nothing alongside what I knew in my heart. I, their mother, had left them.

Karl took an apartment about two blocks away from the town house. The boys would ride their bikes over to see him. They began their own unsubtle form of shuttle diplomacy, trying to get us back together. Sometimes I got sick of hearing about Karl's many virtues. I knew full well what Chris and Luke were up to. I loved them for it.

My career at the newspaper took off. In a matter of months I rose from the newest member of the advertising staff to its director. I was one of the few women, the only one in the Cox newspaper chain, to hold such a post. I did it the only way I knew how—by working harder and longer than anyone else. The more involved I became in the newspaper business, the more I loved it. I wanted to know everything, production, composing, the press room, editorial, and news. I knew I had finally found my niche in the business world, and I was determined to make the most of it.

I wasn't the only one who worked hard. My staff put in nearly as many hours as I did and the sales increase showed it. Haney Womack, who was the general manager, and Chuck Wahlheim accused me of sometimes babying my staff and of sticking up for them when they didn't deserve it. Haney and Chuck were wrong. I was responsible for my department; if my staff needed help, I gave it. If they needed help in their work with other departments, I was there. If they were wrong, they heard about it from me, no one else. When they did something that hurt the paper or sales, they saw something of the kid who learned survival on the streets of Buffalo.

I tried always to be fair and honest with the people who worked for me, and I expected the same thing in return. I could conceive of no other way to treat people. We were friends, we are friends today and will be in the future. I didn't baby my staff; on the contrary, I was a strict boss. That's why they were so productive, and I'll always be proud of that.

I got along well with the other departments at the paper, too, although the road wasn't always smooth. Max Jennings and I kept up a continuous battle. As executive editor, he wanted more space for news. I needed the space for my advertisers. I would preempt his news. Sometimes articles in the news would show my customers in a bad light, fairly and unfairly. We'd argue about it, often with gloves off. Once one of Max's reporters wrote a story about a local merchant who beat up one of his employees and left him hanging by his shirt collar from a hook on the wall. Needless to say, I didn't complain about that story, but the advertiser did come in and take his $50,000 account out of the paper. Usually, the case wasn't so clear-cut and I would speak up. On another occasion we ran a story about choosing the right auto mechanic. Parts of the article implied to me—and to most of the automobile dealers in town—that they were all crooks. I stormed into Max's office and found him with his back up, ready to defend the story. With him sitting down and me standing up on the other side of his desk, we were just about eye to eye. Everyone else left us alone while we slugged it out. I think I won that one. I know I did. He wouldn't admit it, but he wrote a hot memo to the city desk about the story after I left.

Max could be a rough customer, too, but I think he always respected me and the way I battled for my clients and my sales. And I knew, too, that if he had a bad story in the paper, he would feel worse about it than anyone else. Despite our confrontations, or maybe because of what they told us about each other, we became good friends.

The work was hard, every single day, but I loved it.

Not everything was pleasant. One time I had to go into the hospital for two days for minor surgery. I received a bouquet of flowers from one of my salesmen, who signed his name and that of the company he had gone to work for. He had taken his top account, one of the paper's largest, with him. I felt betrayed. I was glad he was gone; he lacked the one quality I prized the most: loyalty. It took me nearly two years to get that account back. I stopped in to see the manager of the drug chain every time I could think of a reason to keep from getting thrown out. I always went with a contract ready for signature. One day I returned to my office and handed Haney the signed contract. The big Texan tried to play the stoic but failed. I had laid $30,000 on his desk. He grinned.

I continued to see Karl, occasionally at first, then once or twice a week. Mostly it was about the kids. It was 1978 and they were teenagers now with all the problems of adolescence. Karl was writing a science fiction novel, the first book in a trilogy, he announced. I asked him if I could read it. I had absolutely no idea this was something Karl had wanted to do. I was mightily curious.

The novel was what I considered to be a truly clever treatise on the nature of power. It concerned a woman who discovers a secret of the past which enables her to rise to universal domination of everything around her. It was good. It really was! As I read, I learned a lot about Karl I hadn't known. There was an imaginative and creative side to him that had escaped me in our twenty years of living together. Now that we were separated, I recognized it.

It was Karl, not I, who was doing something new and constructive above and beyond work. I realized that I had let my work dominate the private side of my life. This made me admire Karl anew, and it helped me recognize what some of our problems had been. There were a lot of things we didn't know about each other. I am confident Karl will sell his book someday, but even if he doesn't, I'll always be grateful for what it taught me about him.

In October of that year, Karl made an important decision which was to turn out to be very wise. He took a new job with a small company just starting out, Comtech Data Corp. This firm wasn't like the ill-fated operation that I had joined when we first moved to Arizona. Karl knew the people who were running it. If they failed, it wouldn't be because of inept management. The firm began to prosper almost immediately. Karl had made the right move.

Karl and I had started to date again. We were a little tentative at first, gingerly testing our relationship. We talked with each other more than we had in years about our jobs, about our plans for the future, about ourselves. We wanted to get back together, something the children also wanted desperately, but we didn't want to remarry only to break up later. Karl and I talked again and again about what had separated us and what we wanted to do with the rest of our lives. The decision was made gradually. A few weeks after Karl had started his new job, I told him, "We're just too ornery to break in anyone else." I took the weekend off—my birthday too—and we flew to Las Vegas. We came back on Monday and went to work, but our relationship was on a new footing. We were happy in a different way. I had thought it over carefully and had made the decision that what I wanted for the rest of my life was to be married to Karl. He told me that when we had married for the first time we hadn't any way of knowing what we were getting into, but after twenty years, the second time around, we knew. He was right. From the new beginning we were more tolerant of one another, more understanding. We had no way of knowing, of course, but our marriage was put back together just in time. I was to need Karl more than I had ever dreamed.

One thing that didn't change after we returned from Las Vegas was my dedication to work. I immediately plunged back into a routine of twelve-hour workdays.

In many respects, the following year would be the happiest of my life. I had the job I had always wanted. Karl and I bought a beautiful new home in a fashionable neighborhood in Mesa. It was a rambling white stucco house with a red-tiled roof. We had sold off most of our furniture when we were divorced, so I had the fun of furnishing my new home. We paid for nearly everything in cash from a balloon payment we received for the house we had owned before we separated.

Again my life was on track, but it was to be one short year before the bottom would fall out of my world once more. In November I went into the hospital for what was diagnosed as pneumonia. I got over the pneumonia, but I was still having trouble breathing. I saw several doctors, including the one who was sure I was suffering from "executive burnout." He was soon proven tragically wrong.

SIX

Several weeks after my visit to Houston, hope was gone. That was the worst period—the only time I was completely in despair. I hid it from Karl for a while, but my own eyes told me unequivocally I would not survive much longer. Still Karl and I delayed telling the children and my mother. It was something we saw no reason to do until it was absolutely necessary.

That time came, for the children, on a hot summer night late in June of 1980. I could hide it no longer; they knew something was wrong. Before dinner that night Karl and I told the kids we wanted to talk to them afterward. The boys were impatient. Chris had a date, and Luke wanted to go across the street to play with a friend.

They squirmed impatiently at the table while Karl cleared the dishes. I began a speech I had rehearsed a hundred times in my mind.

"You know I haven't been feeling well," I began. "Well, it's become more than we have told you up to this point. I have a disease that is rare."

The boys became still.

"It's called primary pulmonary hypertension. The doctor says it's getting out of hand and the medicine is not helping. The trip to Houston didn't help. Nothing has helped. My disease is terminal. I have maybe a year and a half. We don't know."

Chris's jaw became set, the muscles in his face hard. His hands slowly clenched into fists. Karl turned to him and gently put his hand on Chris's arm.

"There is a very real possibility your mother might not be here for your graduation," he said.

I tried to reassure him, my granite-jawed son, by reaching toward him. It was a hollow gesture.

I prayed I could keep my voice steady and calm as I tried to talk to them. "My goal is to survive to see you graduate. All I have at the moment is my will and that goal. I'm going to try to fulfill it as best I can. I'm going to try to live."

Chris said not a word. He looked as if he wanted to break the table in half. I understood his helpless rage—I had felt it myself.

Luke, never the silent one, questioned, "Do you think they might come up with a new medicine?" Then he quickly answered it himself. "Yeah, I'm sure they will, Mom." His questions continued, and he finished with, "You won't die. You'll find a way to make it, Mom."

From that moment, Luke was never to lose hope. He didn't dismiss the gravity of what I had told him, but he had faith in the future. He believed in me more than I did in myself. All through the next months he was to be a source of unwavering comfort and hope.

I looked at my boys in the suddenly quiet room and I wept softly. I felt sorry for the children and I felt sorry for myself. I was sad because Christopher was sitting at the table hurting and there was nothing I could do to relieve his pain. Luke hurt equally but in a different way. I could not help him either. How do you tell your children you are dying?

"Why don't you quit work?" Luke blurted out.

"I need to work. It gives me a sense of reality, a sense of

doing something. You and Chris are at school all day. I can't stay home. What value would it be to stay home then? I feel better if I can accomplish something and be with people."

Luke seemed to understand. Chris remained rigid, fists clenched.

"I want you to go out with your friends and do the things you want to do. Life goes on," I told them. "I don't want you to feel guilty when you leave the house.

"A person is never really dead and gone if you remember them and think of the happy times and not dwell on the sad times. There are a lot of people in the world who have lost parents and who survived and did very well. I don't want you to be bitter."

It was a good speech. I meant every word of it from the bottom of my heart. I knew they wouldn't believe it then. Their faces showed the bitterness they felt. I hoped they would remember later what I said. Maybe it would help when I was gone.

"Well, you're not going to die," Luke insisted.

"That's what I'm hoping too," I said, more brightly than I felt. "Medical science is progressing so fast we can't even keep up with it. There have been more accomplishments in the last fifty years than in all of mankind's history."

That was a cliché, but they seemed to buy it for the moment. Any hope at all, based on any kind of flimsy statement, was better than nothing. I hadn't convinced myself, though.

Still without having said a word, Chris left the table and went to his room. An hour later he came out, got into his car, and raced away, tires screeching. I watched him go and didn't try to stop him. I understood perfectly. For years, when I wanted to think, I had gone driving.

Luke went across the street to play with a friend, Matt Womack, who happened to be the son of my boss. Soon the two of them came over to our house. Matt would not look at me. I could tell that Luke must have shared the news with him.

Karl and I sat and talked quietly, drinking cup after cup of coffee.

"Well, you just can't tell your children you're going to die and make them feel good," I said to Karl.

Karl, ever analytical, agonized over whether we had handled breaking the news to the boys in the best possible way. We talked until we had nothing left to say, and we still had no answer to Karl's question.

Later that night, Chris returned and went directly to his room. I waited a few minutes and went to him. He was sobbing. I put my arms around him, remembering when he was a small child. If it rained, I was supposed to stop it. He had thought I could do anything. I wanted him to still have that simple faith in me, but the years had robbed him of that. I had told him I was going to die. He was helpless and without hope. His heart was breaking and mine with it. I sat with my arms around him for a long time.

After that I threw myself into work with every ounce of strength I could muster. Somehow survival had become linked in my mind with my ability to keep working. To quit work was a step down the road toward death. As the hot summer dragged by, I knew I was losing the fight. I was growing weaker and weaker. Every day it was harder just to get out of bed and get dressed. Once I got to work, I usually had a rush of energy and felt better for a while. But now the rush didn't last very long. Only a few people in the office knew the extent of my rapid deterioration. Haney Womack and John Hanron knew and did what they could to help. My secretary Carole Doyle and Joyce Howland, a close friend and one of my salespeople, both shared my fears, or at least those I was willing to share with them. But even though I wanted to talk about what was happening to me, it was absolutely impossible to express how I felt. No one else had any frame of reference for understanding what was happening to me. Again and again, I was in anguish because I was so lonely. But dying is something you do alone.

A new facet of my disease began to manifest itself, one that bothered me even more than the constant weariness. It was becoming difficult to remember things. The inadequate supply of oxygen reaching my brain had started to affect my mind.

The constant fatigue began to dominate my life. There was never any pain, simply an enormous burden of tiredness. I felt it to the very core of my being.

One day I was especially tired and went home earlier than usual, about 1:30 in the afternoon. I changed into a comfortable hostess gown and lay down for an hour or so, taking oxygen from the tall green tank alongside my bed. After I had rested a few minutes and had taken the oxygen, I felt better and decided to read the *Tribune.* One article caught my eye; something inside me came to attention. I sat up and clutched the paper tighter, rereading the story. It told of Dr. Bruce Reitz and his work on heart-lung transplants with rhesus monkeys at Stanford. The story, on an inside page of the *Tribune,* mentioned that Dr. Reitz would soon be looking for human candidates for the surgery.

I sat and thought about it for a while. Several years earlier I had read the book *Hearts* by Thomas Thompson. It was the story of the early years of heart transplant surgery and the doctors who were involved. In an appendix to the book was a list of transplant recipients, how many of them survived and the name of the surgeon who had performed the transplant. Opposite the names of those people still living, one name was conspicuously repeated: Dr. Norman Shumway of Stanford University Medical Center.

At the time I told Karl, "If I ever need a transplant, I'd go to Stanford." I recalled those words with a feeling of bitter irony.

That evening, Joyce Howland and John Hanron, my ever-loyal friends, called me to be sure I had seen the story. John added, "Mary, this is something you ought to look into." His deep voice carried a hint of hope. I agreed with him.

The next time I went to see Dr. Slater, I told him about the story and the work at Stanford and asked him what he thought.

The doctor just shook his head and smiled. He clearly did not want to encourage my desperate dreaming. "I think it's very interesting" is all I could get him to say. He did not offer any encouragement.

The days dragged by. I hadn't thought it possible to feel more tired. I was wrong. More than ever I was weary. More than ever I was without hope. Always ahead of me was the same darkening horizon. Still I had to try any chance. If there was one legacy I wanted to leave my children, it was that, win or lose, as long as I was alive I had tried.

By September I was so weak it was all I could do to drive the few miles from my home to my office. One day in September, as I lay on the bed taking my oxygen, I was aware of a cold feeling deep in my bones, a feeling that had been growing for weeks. I had noticed it before, but now I knew what it was; it was the way death feels when it approaches. I thought again of the article about Dr. Bruce Reitz. It had been on my mind almost constantly since I first read it. I decided to act.

Just to lift the phone alongside the bed was a major effort, but my mind was made up. I was going to try.

I wasn't sure exactly where Stanford was located, near San Francisco was all I knew. I called the Mesa Public Library. The librarian told me where Stanford was and gave me the phone number. In a few minutes I had reached the cardiovascular unit.

Joanie Miller, the head nurse in the transplant unit, took the call. I plunged in.

"I'm Mary Gohlke from Mesa, Arizona. I read an article a while back about Dr. Reitz and his research on monkeys and heart-lung transplants. The article said he would be looking for candidates. I think I may be one."

Joanie said nothing. I continued.

"I would very much like to talk to Dr. Reitz if he has the time."

Joanie Miller probed gently.

"What do you have?"

"Pulmonary hypertension."

"Is it primary?"

"Yes," I answered.

"Just a minute," Joanie said.

The next voice I heard was that of Bruce Reitz.

"May I help you?"

The voice I heard was gentle and friendly. There was more; some quality in his voice made the offer of help more than just a conventional greeting. He sounded . . . well, just genuine. My "gut feeling" was a good one.

I began at the beginning, quickly sketching my medical history. He listened patiently.

"I read about you in the newspaper where I work," I finished.

"What do you do?" Dr. Reitz asked.

I explained about my job, then changed the subject back to the reason I had called. "How can I qualify for a transplant?"

Dr. Reitz answered with a question of his own.

"How have you been feeling?"

I told him of my extreme weariness ending with, "I'm still working a couple of hours a day, but I can't do that much longer."

"Have you had a heart catheterization which confirms the diagnosis?" Dr. Reitz asked.

"Yes," I told him, adding, "I've been to see Dr. DeBakey at Houston too and it was confirmed there."

"What have you been told about the future?" he continued.

"In March my doctor said I had about five years, but the disease is progressing more rapidly than was expected at first. Now they tell me I'm lucky if I have a year to live. That's why I would like to be a candidate for a transplant."

"What makes you think you'd like to be a candidate?" Bruce seemed to ignore the reason I had given. In my heart I knew what he wanted to know. He didn't want my medical opinion. He wanted to know why I wanted a transplant. I have a saying I always gave to my salespeople when they were having trouble closing a contract. "When all else fails, try honesty." I decided to take my own advice.

"I don't want to die."

It was the answer Bruce Reitz wanted to hear. We discussed what my Arizona doctors had told me.

"I just feel time's awasting," I concluded. "I want to do something."

"All right," Dr. Reitz said. "Have your doctor send me your medical records and send me his phone number. I'll get back to you."

Before our conversation ended, I had one more question I wanted to ask.

"How many candidates are you looking for this year—to do the heart-lung transplant?"

"I'd like to do ten," Dr. Reitz answered.

"Well," I said, "I'd like to be number ten. I'd like to see how the rest of them turn out. I'd rather you had a little more practice first."

Bruce Reitz chuckled. He said he'd like to meet me.

When I hung up the phone, I had hope again. Maybe I took unreasonable comfort from the kindness in Dr. Reitz's voice, but God, I needed something to hang onto.

Suddenly I started to smile. In truth, I was awfully pleased with myself. I had just made an extraordinarily important sales call, and I felt I was about to clinch a deal. It was an instinct that seldom led me wrong. I felt happier than I had in a long time.

The minute Karl came through the door that evening I gave him the news. I told him I had hope again. I didn't know whether I would be accepted or not. I didn't know if I could be helped by a transplant. I didn't know whether or not my life could be saved. There was a lot I didn't know. I only knew I had found hope. Karl said little. He just put his arms around me and gave me a hug. He was taciturn, but I knew his spirits were lifted. I had found a chance for a solution other than dying.

The next day was my regular appointment with Dr. Slater. When I told him what I had done and that Dr. Reitz wanted to see my records, he was cooperative but unenthusiastic.

"The agony will not be worth the ecstasy," he told me.

I bristled. Dr. Slater wasn't me; he wasn't dying. From his point of view, he was doing all he could, but he wasn't going to take even a long shot away from me. Not ever! I felt Dr. Slater had sympathy, but no real understanding of what I was going through. As usual, I left his office feeling worse than when I had arrived. He had poured cold water on the embers of my hopes again by telling me I had no choice other than slow death, that the risk of transplant surgery was too great. I disagreed violently; my other choice carried no risk at all. It was death! My determination was not diminished in the least by Dr. Slater's pessimism. To the contrary, Slater had lent me resolve. I vowed to put him behind me as fast as I could. Dr. Reitz was the only one to give me hope, and indeed it was more than anyone else had offered me in a long time.

Dr. Slater had been right about one thing, though. As I made my weekly visits to him, he marveled at how rapidly my disease was progressing. Both Karl and I knew my race against the clock had started long ago. We wondered how many months really remained to me. A few weeks earlier I had started to suffer blackouts. The first time it happened, Karl called Dr. Slater immediately. The doctor told him the truth; nothing could be done. The blackouts were a normal manifestation of my disease. My heart was failing. Either I would come out of the blackouts or I wouldn't. It was one way primary pulmonary hypertension victims often died. They would just go into a coma and never make it back. After the first few times I passed out, Karl knew exactly how to handle things. He would lay me down with my feet elevated and watch. I often have wondered about the hell he must have gone through during those times. He told me that when I was out I always kept one finger moving, the index finger of my left hand. He'd sit beside me and watch that finger move. He has never told me what he was thinking as he sat there. I know he was pulling for me. Maybe it was as much his will as mine that sustained that twitch of life. We'll never know.

During my visit to the cardiologist after my first blackout, Slater's partner Dr. Paul Simmons went through his examination and then patiently explained to Karl and me why I was weakening so fast. It was the same straightforward message both doctors had given us in various versions before.

Karl was numbed anew. We drove to a nearby coffee shop and ordered breakfast. Karl began what must have been the toughest conversation of his life. He reached across the table and took my hand.

"What arrangements do you want me to make?" he asked.

"What do you mean?"

"Do you want to be buried here or in Buffalo?" He started to cry, oblivious of everyone around us. I, too, began to weep softly. Karl had never given up faith, but now he had to face the very real possibility that I would die. He saw that his hopes might be disappointed. I squeezed his hand gently.

"Here. I want to be buried here," I said. "I just want a memorial service. No matter what my family says. No matter what anyone says. That's what I want. I don't want all those dumb remarks made over my coffin."

I had always thought it ridiculous for people to stand beside a coffin and say how natural or well the deceased looked. I had considered cremation, but something Luke had said as a little boy made up my mind. He had told me that if I were cremated he wouldn't be able to visit my grave.

I squeezed Karl's hand, still startled by the tears streaming down his face. It was the first time I had ever seen him cry. How I had underestimated the pain I was causing him!

"After I'm gone, I want you to take the kids on a trip for a few weeks. Just be with the boys. They will be hurting. They'll need to be close to you. Whatever you do, don't refuse to talk about it."

Karl nodded. The tears filled my eyes, but I was determined to be very objective.

"The boys will feel bad and they won't want to talk to you about it because you'll feel bad. Everybody needs to let their grief out. Promise me you won't get into a 'Don't talk about mother' habit. I think talking will help all of you get through that bad period of time."

Karl nodded agreement.

It wasn't a happy conversation, but as we left the coffee shop, I was glad we had had it. I was dying. It was very real to me and I wanted to talk about it. I wanted to know that when I was gone, my family and our world wouldn't fall apart. I needed assurance that my loved ones would be all right when I could do no more. Talking helped relieve the terrible loneliness I felt.

SEVEN

I COULD NO LONGER GO ON. THE TIME HAD FINALLY ARRIVED when I had to quit work. My mind wanted to continue, but my body said no.

For months I had fought to keep working. It was now more than four months since Michael DeBakey had sent me home to die. Karl and I had often discussed what we would do when I could no longer work. Most of all, I feared to stay home alone—just waiting to die. I also worried about our finances. We lived comfortably, well within our means, but I knew the loss of my income would hurt, more than hurt. I wondered how we would get along. Karl repeatedly told me not to worry, he'd find a way. I wondered if he would or if he was just trying to hide one more worry from me.

I had hoped to work until at least the end of the year. Part of my pay was in the form of a year-end bonus based on sales. I knew sales had been good for the nine months I had worked. I had hoped my bonus would be enough to carry us through the bad times ahead. It would be six months before I would get my first disability check, which would amount to less than my normal weekly earnings. And I would never see the bonus.

I went to see Charlie Wahlheim, the publisher of the paper, and we decided my last day of work would be the end of the pay week, Thursday, September 10. I hated that conversation with Charlie. What we were really saying to each other, and to everyone, was that from that day forward I would never work again.

Wahlheim threw a late afternoon party for me at the restaurant of a nearby hotel, inviting my closest friends from the newspaper and the senior executives. It was a lousy party.

"How do you give a party for someone going off to die?" someone asked Max Jennings, the editor. A long time later, he would tell me about that.

I arrived early. It was almost too warm to be sitting outside next to the swimming pool. The surroundings were pleasant. I wished the circumstances were half as pleasant. I took a chair under an umbrella as my friends began to arrive. It was apparent to everyone that they were saying good-bye before the funeral. I was the corpse, able to see and hear but just as helpless. I felt sorry for those who came. I knew that by showing up they were saying they really cared. Yet, there was nothing for them to say. Some people wandered over to tell me how well I looked. It was not true. They knew it. I knew it. Anyone who could see knew it! I looked like a dying woman: my eyes were dull and sunken; it took all my strength just to sit in a chair and smile. There were few smiling faces at that party. One who didn't smile was the supervisor of the pressroom, Norm Miller. A big bear of a man, Norm was most often seen working around his three-story press, covered with ink and yelling instructions like the captain of a tugboat. He looked out of place and uncomfortable in slacks and a sport shirt. He and I had had more than one shouting match over problems at the paper. I imagine we made a curious pair when we battled, little five foot me standing almost against him, looking up, waving what I considered a poor piece of printing in his face. Norm would tower over me and yell back his version of what had gone wrong. We learned to work together. We argued but we got along. I gained an understanding of some of Norm's problems, and I think he had grown to admire the tough little woman who was never afraid to let him know her thoughts.

He walked over to me at the party and said not a word He didn't try to smile. We looked at each other for a mo ment, and he reached down and put his big arms around me and hugged me to him. When he pulled his face away, I was startled to see he had tears in his eyes. I was happy for a moment that he had come. Then I was sad again. I didn't want to say good-bye to Norm; I didn't want to hurt him, but I was.

People left the party as soon as they could. There was nothing anyone could say to add a note of optimism. They were helpless in front of me and I knew I was morose.

That night I shared my thoughts with Karl. "I felt so bad for everyone else there," I told him. It was so sad. Had I been a guest, I wouldn't have known what to say either.

Karl looked at me and said levelly, "Well, maybe we can have another party next year—when you come home."

His words startled me for a moment, then I knew what he was thinking about: my call to Dr. Reitz at Stanford, the transplant. I knew Karl had never lost hope, and now he had something concrete to hang on to. It was only a thread, but it was hope. I hadn't yet even been accepted as a candidate. We didn't know if a transplant would help me. Still I knew Karl was optimistic. He's a hidebound realist, but he has a saying, "When you've only got two chances—slim and none—take slim."

His optimism infected me. I felt better, at least for the moment.

The next day began my long wait. I had always loved to read, but my illness made reading difficult and unpleasant. I had trouble concentrating and lost my place frequently. I tired quickly, just from the effort of holding a book. I didn't like my first day away from work, not at all.

I talked regularly with Dr. Reitz. Sometimes I called him; sometimes he called me. Our telephone conversation was often the high point of my day. In a macabre waiting game, we both had to hold off until I was truly near death. Because of the experimental nature of the operation and the very real risk that I would not survive it, Bruce was bound by moral duty to make sure that he was not asking me to sacrifice needlessly whatever quality time I had left, in the event that I were to die.

I was running out of time. No one had to tell me or Karl. My blackouts were becoming more frequent. I could no longer drive. It was too dangerous. I told Dr. Reitz what was happening to me, and after one particularly bad blackout, Dr. Reitz said I'd better come up to Stanford. He wanted to examine me. I would also be interviewed as a prospective candidate for a heart-lung transplant.

On October 12, 1980, Karl and I drove to the airport in Phoenix. I was so weak that I rode in a wheelchair to the plane door and was carried on. I was on oxygen most of the time, and Karl was worried about the lack of oxygen in the plane cabin at higher altitudes. He called the airline and they assured him the plane was pressurized to low altitude. Also in an emergency, oxygen would be available.

In Palo Alto, we checked into a Holiday Inn near the Stanford Medical Center. We dined at the motel and went to bed soon after. Our appointment the next morning was scheduled at an early hour. I was exhausted from the trip, but I was excited. I felt this was really going to be it—the same intuition I'd sensed the first time I had talked to Bruce Reitz on the phone. The awareness that I might not be accepted made me nervous, but I had an idea of what they were looking for: someone who would fight, who wanted to live, who had a reason to live. I made up my mind that if nothing else, I would leave Bruce Reitz with the impression that I was a fighter. I might not make it, but I was going to give it one hell of a try.

The next morning I registered as an outpatient and was interviewed by a young clerk who asked why I was there.

"I'm being interviewed for a heart-lung transplant," I said.

"A heart and lung?" the startled clerk asked. "Both?"

"Yes."

The clerk slowly wrote the information down. I had the distinct impression she thought I didn't know what I was talking about. She made no comment, however; just issued my little outpatient card and directed me to where I should go.

Karl wheeled me upstairs to a chilly waiting room where we sat for a few minutes before we were led down a long hallway where a sign said Eye Clinic.

"Eye Clinic?" I asked Karl. He laughed.

"Where the hell is the transplant clinic?" We laughed. I found out later there is no such sign anywhere in the Stanford Medical Center. I guess it isn't necessary to show transplant patients the way around. They learn it themselves all too well.

The tests began. I was given an ECG, and an X ray was taken. The nurse administered the whole battery of tests with which I was all too familiar. Finally we were ushered into a tiny examining room. The nurse took my temperature and blood pressure, then left. Karl and I sat alone in the tiny cubicle, trying to make conversation. The attempt was an abysmal failure. We were incredibly preoccupied with what was to come.

Lois Christopherson, a member of the transplant evaluation team, entered first. Lois was trained in social work and did her best to put me at ease. She couldn't possibly have succeeded. This was to be the most important interview of my life. It *was* my life. I didn't know what the "right" answers were, so I decided to be honest.

Yet as Lois and I talked, I began to relax. I sat on the edge of the examining table and we talked of my family, my children, my hopes and fears. Her questions posed no surprises. I relaxed a little.

The door opened and Bruce Reitz entered the room. I looked him in the eye and he looked back, a calm steady gaze. I've never liked people who won't look you in the eye, so his response reassured me at once. He walked over and shook my hand, placing his other hand on top of mine. His handshake was firm and gentle. I decided I liked this man; more than that, I trusted him. I felt better.

"Well, I'm here," I said. "I'm glad to meet you."

"I'm glad to meet you, Mary," he said gently. He was a slender, balding man in his mid-thirties. My first thought was that he looked kind. I thought it amusing that he wore penny loafers. I later found out that he never wore any other kind of shoe; it was characteristic of his casual style.

As I looked at this man my vague hope underwent a transformation. The idea of a heart-lung transplant had never seemed quite real before. It was something you read in a newspaper, something that took place far away and involved other people. Now, Bruce Reitz could make it real. I had more than a hope. I had a chance.

After Reitz excused himself for being late (no doctor had ever apologized to me before), the interview continued. Lois came to what I sensed were the crucial questions.

"Why do you want this operation?" she asked.

"Because I want to live."

"What do you mean by that? What is living to you?"

"I want to live a quality life. I want to be able to eventually go back to work. I want to be able to enjoy my family. I have two sons to raise and the job is not done yet. I don't want to be a vegetable lying in bed. I want to be able to get back into life. I want to live, whether it's for five minutes, five days, or five years. I want to live without feeling the way I feel now. I want to be able to live, to breathe, to feel good." It was the longest speech I had made about myself in a long time.

For Karl, Lois obviously was interested in what kind of support he would be able to provide me when push came to shove. The questions were not difficult or hard, but again and again, both interviewers hammered at that point. Once she asked him, "What if it doesn't work? What if she dies?"

Said Karl simply, "I think I would grieve for the rest of my life. But I would raise the boys, and I would go on with my life, because you have to do that." He told me later he knew he had given a good answer because Lois seemed to relax. Her body language told him she had had one of her concerns resolved.

Immediately, Bruce and Lois began to paint the downside of the operation. They weren't being negative, but they wanted both Karl and me to know what I was getting into, to know the ways in which the transplant would permanently change my life.

"You may be cured of your present disease, Mary, but there will be other factors, problems you will have to live with," Reitz warned. "Your body will try to reject the transplanted organs, and you will have to take certain medications to prevent rejection. These same medications suppress your immune systems, which, in turn, means you'll always be more susceptible to infection."

Karl, ever interested in the technical aspects of everything, asked, "Won't her body accept the new heart and lungs in time?"

Bruce shook his head. "No. While the body does build up a certain degree of tolerance, you"—he looked directly at me—"will have to take these medications for the rest of your life.

"The most important drug is cyclosporin A, which suppresses one of the body's mechanisms that fights infection—the mechanism it suppresses is the one that also causes rejection.

"You'll have to take other things as well, the most important of which is prednisone, a steroid. Unfortunately, these drugs have side effects. Cyclosporin can cause cancer. Prednisone tends to make your bones brittle and make you into a bleeder. There are several other drugs you will have to take as well."

I was beginning to feel a little confused. I think the doctor sensed it because he changed the subject.

"We'll go over these matters later, after we've seen whether you'd make a good candidate for a transplant and before you make your final decision.

"The most important thing for you to understand is that the heart-lung transplant is an experimental operation. It was tried three times before—not at Stanford—and none of the attempts succeeded. The patient who survived longest lived twenty-three days. The main problem so far has been the antirejection drugs, which interfere with the body's ability to heal. The trachea is particularly slow to heal, and eventually infection sets in. Our work with the monkeys leads us to believe that with cyclosporin A that problem can be overcome."

I felt an intense concern about the welfare of the monkeys.

"How are the monkeys doing?" I asked.

Bruce smiled. "Very well; one, named Momma, has lived fourteen months since the transplant, which is quite long in human terms."

He sobered again. "I want you to understand that the results with monkeys are not the same as what will happen to a human. We have nothing sure to go on. We think that the results will be similar to those of a heart transplant; but I want you to realize this operation is not the same"—he emphasized the words *not the same*—"as a heart transplant and I can't tell you exactly what the risk is.

"I can tell you that a heart transplant recipient has about a 70 percent chance of living a year and about a fifty-fifty chance of living five years. The outlook for recipients has steadily been improving, and we hope their chances will be better in the future. Still, I can't give you any guarantee. Here and now that is the risk—and only if a heart-lung result is the same as a heart transplant. I think it will be, but at present I can't even promise you that."

My mind was racing. The picture being painted about my future wasn't pretty. I realized he wasn't trying to make a transplant sound pleasant; it wouldn't be. He was describing a hard reality. He wanted me to know what I was getting into. I decided I liked him even more than I had thought.

Karl and Lois left the room. I changed into a hospital gown for my first examination. Reitz listened carefully to my heart and lungs, and his opinion was quickly formed.

"I see no reason to do another heart catheterization," he said. "The one Dr. Simmons did confirms your disease. I know Paul and he did a good job."

I wasn't disappointed by Dr. Reitz's decision. I didn't look forward to another catheterization. He then told me something else less cheering.

"We're not ready to do surgery now. We don't have approval from the FDA to use cyclosporin A as yet. We hope to soon, possibly within a few weeks."

His next statement could have made only someone in my situation feel encouraged.

"A transplant is done only as a last-ditch measure, when all other methods have been exhausted and when you cannot reasonably expect to live more than six months. You are not quite ready for a transplant yet. You are too healthy."

"Fine," I told him. "I'd like to be number ten anyhow, after you've got your act together and everything straightened out."

Bruce smiled in response. He left for a moment while I dressed, then he came back and closed the door of the tiny room. We stood looking at each other for a few seconds and he took my hand. "Mary, we're going to make it. I feel right about it."

I recalled an article I had once read by a psychologist whose name I can't remember. In it, he said that true insight with another individual is one of the most powerful experiences known to man, but that instances of true communication are few and far between, totalling not more than thirty seconds in a lifetime. I felt that way about Bruce Reitz at that moment. I believed then he would give me a new life and I would give him the opportunity to carry out a successful transplant, the one thing he had spent five years of research to achieve. We stood for a few moments more after he had spoken, just looking at each other.

Lois Christopherson and Karl rejoined us. Dr. Reitz left and Lois took Karl and me to the North Intensive Care Unit where I would be if and when I had a transplant. In one of the isolation rooms a man was sitting on the edge of the bed, enjoying his lunch.

"This patient received his new heart eight days ago," Lois told us. I looked at the man sitting there, relaxed, eating. "God," I thought to myself, "wouldn't it be wonderful to be able to just sit and calmly have dinner again." Eating even a small meal had become an exhausting experience.

Before we left, Lois made an unexpected request.

"I'd like you to sit down and write a short personal history for me," she asked. "Write down your interests, your likes and dislikes."

"Why?" I was puzzled.

Lois smiled. "If you become a transplant recipient, you'll spend a long time here. Your nurses will be with you twenty-four hours a day. We try to have nurses who are compatible with you, who share some of your interests. There will be enough to get on your nerves without adding to it."

Lois spoke as we stood in one of the transplant rooms, which was unoccupied at the time. It was a white sterile room crowded with a bewildering display of machines and instruments. The windows looked out on a serene scene of trees and lawn. It seemed like a nice room. I didn't know then that I would spend nearly three months of my life in that very room. The day would come when I would grow to hate it.

"In one way," Lois continued, "you'll be a nice change. Most of our transplant recipients are men, you know." She hastened to add, "Serious heart problems are much more common among men than among women at an age when a transplant will do the most good." I think, like many people, she expected me to be a women's libber because I had been successful in the business world. I'm not, but I've always believed that if you work and are good at your job you can get ahead. If you can't do it where you are, go elsewhere. Let those hidebound by their own prejudices fail on their own; why help them?

Karl and I left and went back to the motel. I was exhausted by the day's activities. We would leave for home the following day.

I lay down for a rest, and the events of the day kept running through my mind. I had been promised nothing. Dr. Reitz could not have accepted me as a candidate on his own wish alone. Transplant candidates were selected by a committee that reviewed the medical tests and interviews. At the time, I didn't know how they did it. I didn't really care. Most of what I'd been told sounded unpleasant at best. I knew one thing, however. The people at Stanford were caring and competent; they stood between me and death.

As I drifted off to sleep, I remembered Bruce Reitz's remark that they didn't have permission as yet to use cyclosporin A. I felt a twinge of worry, but shrugged it off. The statement didn't mean much to me then. Little did I know that in a few short months my life would hang precariously in the balance because of that problem, which seemed so soluble at the time.

EIGHT

TEN DAYS AFTER OUR INTERVIEW AT STANFORD, BRUCE REITZ called me. "We're going to do this, Mary," he said. "You've been accepted as a candidate."

My heart, diseased or not, was full of happiness I smiled when I told Karl, and he chuckled at me.

"Honey," he said, "Do you realize we're sitting here happy at the news that you're going to be almost literally cut in half, have two major organs taken out and replaced, go through God knows what, and then be on medication for the rest of your life?"

"But there will be a rest of my life," I said. Tears filled my eyes. They were happy tears. "I'm going to make it, Karl. I know I will."

He put his hand tenderly on my arm. "I know you will, Mary."

One cloud remained. Stanford still didn't have approval to use cyclosporin A for the heart-lung transplant. I resisted the temptation to call Stanford every day. Instead, I called about every two weeks. Each time I was told that the request for approval to use cyclosporin was being processed through channels. I understood that the holdup was a delay in approval from the Food and Drug Administration. After each of these conversations I was both encouraged and disappointed. I realized that people were standing by to help, but I was increasingly frustrated with the bureaucracy that would not let me have the drug I needed to live. My friends could sense my frustration—I guess I told them about it, too. They did everything they could. They would order lunch at a restaurant in advance, sweep by, and get me. We would have a happy, busy lunch that never seemed to last long enough. Sometimes some of the bunch at the *Tribune* would bring lunch to my house so we could eat together.

I felt like doing little else. I was in no pain, but the weariness became a little more pronounced each day. I often thought that I could get no weaker than I already was, but I was wrong. The weariness seemed to be settling into my very bones. I spent more and more time in bed taking oxygen. It helped a little.

I continued to see my cardiologist in Phoenix. It did not do much good. All Dr. Slater could tell me was that my health was deteriorating rapidly, and I certainly needed no one to tell me that. My visits to the doctor did provide me with mild amusement on one point. Dr. Slater's attitude toward the heart-lung transplant began to change. I don't know what accounted for his new optimism—maybe I'd made him look into it more, maybe he talked to Stanford about transplants. Still, I no longer heard "The agony won't be worth the ecstasy." I guess I've never forgiven him for that statement. How could he possibly be in a position to judge!

About the only thing I really had to do besides wait for the cyclosporin approval was to figure out how to tell my mother what was going on.

In August, before Karl and I had gone to Stanford, I knew I could no longer put off telling her. Still, I couldn't decide the best way to do it. One evening, sitting at home, I reached for the phone on impulse and called her. Mother lived in Florida and used to come out and see us once or twice a year. I had hoped to wait until her next visit and tell her face to face, but that night I knew I couldn't wait any longer.

We exchanged family small talk for a few minutes, then I broke the news.

"Mother, you know I haven't been feeling well," I began.

"Still!" Mother interrupted. "What does your doctor say? Maybe you had better get a new one. It seems to me you've been sick a long time now."

I answered her first question. It hurt to say it. "Mother, I'm dying."

There were a few moments of silence, then Mother asked, "Are you sure? Did Karl talk to the doctor?"

"Yes, Mother, I'm sure," I said. "And Karl did talk to the doctor." Mother has always had a high regard for Karl's opinion. Nothing is a fact until he says so. I'm not demeaning Karl's intelligence—he's probably the smartest human being I've ever known—but I did think I knew enough to understand the doctor when he said I was dying. I think Mother, however, regards Karl with a little awe. If he says it's so—it's so.

"I'll come out there," Mother stated with an air of finality.

"Mother, it's not necessary. There is really nothing you can do. Besides, you can't quit your job."

I'd said the wrong words. There were things she could do and she knew it.

"Who's doing the cooking and cleaning and taking care of the house?" she asked.

"I do some," I said. "Karl does most of it and the kids help."

"Karl has to work. He's tired when he gets home. I'll come out."

I didn't bother to point out that she had worked all her life and still had cooked and taken care of a house. It would have been pointless. Mother comes from a generation in which men didn't do housework.

Mother decided to come out in early September, but

six days before she was to leave Florida, she fell at work and broke her knee. It was November before she arrived, painfully hobbling along with a walker.

We slipped into a routine of quiet lethargy. I spent much of the time in bed taking oxygen, trying to build up as much strength as I could so I could spend time with Karl and the boys in the evenings. But I was so terribly weak that some nights I could only walk out to say hello and maybe watch television with them for a few minutes before I had to go back to bed. I slept fitfully during the day and at night. One day I realized I was deteriorating mentally as well as physically. It was another brutal twist I hated. My sense of humor was gone. Or maybe I just didn't have enough energy to laugh any more. It made no difference.

December came and I called Dr. Reitz. Stanford still didn't have approval for the cyclosporin. I was irked and growing more insistent.

"What's holding it up?" I demanded. "Don't they know I'm getting sicker?"

Bruce Reitz was as puzzled as I was. For the umpteenth time, he assured me that he and Stanford were doing everything they could. I was not impressed and Reitz knew it.

"Well, when I get to Stanford, I'm going to teach you how to be a street fighter," I told him. Bruce chuckled.

Christmas came and went. It was meaningless to my family. It was difficult for anyone to forget, even for a moment, that I was dying rapidly. I wanted so badly for it to be a merry Christmas. It might be my last, and I wanted everyone to remember it as a happy time. They all tried, but their efforts were pathetic. I cried a lot on Christmas Day.

Early in January, Karl and I went to see Dr. Slater, who examined me again. By then the doctor who had first told me I was certain to die had done a complete about-face!

"What are they doing out there?" he demanded, anger

in his voice. "Why don't they get this transplant going? We don't have much time left."

I had missed it, but Slater's opinion about the transplant had become so favorable that now "we" were having the transplant. I had never forgiven him for cutting me off from all hope, even as bizarre a solution as a double transplant. He had not assisted me in seeking the transplant nor had he encouraged me once I had told him about my decision to visit Stanford. I wasn't going to let him forget it. I looked him in the eye.

"What's this 'we' shit?" I said levelly. "It wasn't your decision. It was mine. You were the guy who didn't want me to do it, remember?" He had nothing to say.

Maybe I was hard on him, but he had hurt me when I needed encouragement and I was angry and incredibly frustrated over the cyclosporin problem. Things were never again quite the same between us.

By the first week in February I was so weak that some days it took all my will just to turn over in bed. The weariness simply enveloped me. There was little I could do. Mercifully, there was no pain, but that was little consolation.

Several times I slipped into unconsciousness. Everyone in the family knew that sooner or later I simply would not pull out of one of those blackouts. The worst part for Karl was the flat statement from my doctors that it would serve little purpose for him to summon the local paramedics during those spells. Either I would come out of it or I wouldn't. I suffered one blackout during the Christmas holidays and two more during January. Each time I was unconscious several minutes.

Near the middle of February, on President's Day, Karl brought me a cup of tea and I sat up in bed and talked to him while he got ready for work. A young woman, Kathy Nelson, who came to clean once a week, bounced in cheerily and worked efficiently through the house. Mother had progressed to a cane but still could not do much housework. I got up for a little while but went back to bed after Karl left. Mother came into my bedroom to ask me something. I heard her, but she sounded so far away. I could not answer. "I'm going," I said.

It was the same phrase I always used when blacking out.

"Kathy, call Karl!" Mother screamed. That was the last thing I remember. They made no move to call the paramedics. Karl raced home, but by the time he got there, I was coming out of it. Mother sat beside me and watched the index finger on my left hand, calling my name softly. I still don't quite understand it, but I always managed to keep that finger moving when I was out. It was as if I still had some control, even when I was unconscious.

When Karl got home, he continued to call my name quietly.

"Can you hear me?" Karl asked. "Wake up, Mary. Wake up."

The first thing I said when I recovered enough to talk was "How long have I been out?"

"A good while, this time. I think about twenty-five minutes," Karl said.

I was angry.

"Why is it taking so long?" I asked no one in particular. "I'll be dead before I get there." I did not need to explain where. I knew this time I was slipping fast. Karl made me a cup of tea. When he came back, I ordered: "Get the telephone."

I called Dr. Reitz.

"I've just had another blackout, a bad one," I told him. "When am I going to be able to come to Stanford? I'm afraid. For the first time I'm really afraid that I'm running out of time."

Bruce Reitz was gentle with me. I could hear the pain and exasperation in his voice. "Well, Mary, we still haven't received permission from the FDA."

"That's crazy," I told him. It was the exact conversation

we had had so many times. "They've approved it for heart transplants, why not heart-lung transplants?"

"I agree with you, Mary. We've done everything we can to get it going."

"I'm tired of holding on. I'm dying and I don't like it. What are the logical reasons?"

"Mary, I agree with you," Bruce said. "I know what you're feeling and I don't blame you."

"How long do you think it's going to be?"

"Mary, I hate to tell you this. I feel bad about it, but I think it's going to be at least another five to ten weeks."

I felt as if I had ice packed around me. Somehow I was calm. "To hell with protocol," I said to myself.

"I don't think I've got ten weeks," I said aloud. "I'm afraid I may not even have five weeks."

"All I can tell you is hang in there. We're going to get this done," Bruce said.

I hung up the phone and sat for a few minutes, crying softly. "Five weeks, ten weeks, what the hell is going on?" I asked no one. "Then I will still have to wait for a donor." The anger had subsided while I talked to Bruce, but now it welled up inside me again, stronger than before.

"I think some bureaucrat's neglect is going to determine whether I live or die," I exploded. "I feel someone hasn't done his paperwork and I'm a file on somebody's desk."

Karl could only nod agreement. I stopped crying. I'd spent enough tears. I did what I've always done. I had to act. I picked up the telephone and began to dial.

"Who are you calling?" Karl asked.

"I'm calling Max," I said. Max was Max Jennings, executive editor of the *Mesa Tribune.* I had worked with him long enough to know he might have an idea. I knew he had the ability to get his hands on information quickly. Perhaps he could help.

Max grabbed the phone on the second ring. There were no greetings.

"Max, do you know who the head of the FDA is?"

I know he was shocked at the sound of my voice. It sounded faint, and old. He was used to the woman who would argue him flat with the voice and vocabulary of a dockworker. I knew he was sitting there, leaning forward, his elbows on the desk, making sure he caught every word as he always did when he was paying attention.

"No, but I can find out in a hurry," he said. "Why?"

"I'm out of time. I can't wait any longer. My doctor tells me it's going to be another five to ten weeks before I get the cyclosporin. Max, I'm not going to be here that long. I'm dying. Can you get me the FDA guy's name?"

We had worked together long enough for histrionics to be unnecessary. He didn't say anything for a moment. When he did I could hear the tears in his voice.

"You've got it," Max said. "I'll be back to you in a half an hour."

Max had interviewed me sometime earlier and was sitting on the story about my selection as the first person in years to receive a heart-and-lung transplant. The operation had been attempted three times several years before. All the patients died quickly. Max explained to me that it would be a big story. I thought he was exaggerating, but I had no problems with the interview. He told me he wouldn't print it until I went to Stanford because he was sure the media would drive me crazy. I thought he was being overly dramatic, but I was willing for him to write the story in whichever way he wanted. He was right about one thing. I had no idea when I was accepted as a candidate that I would be the one to go first. But I knew now that if I underwent the operation at all, it would be Reitz's first on a human being. If I waited for him to operate on the other candidates, I wouldn't be around when my turn came. Both Lois Christopherson, the Stanford social worker, and Bruce had warned us there would be a lot of media interest. Karl didn't believe it.

After my call to him, Max knew the shape I was in. He knew me well enough to know I was desperate. Predictably, he reacted as would any good newsman chasing a good story on deadline. He had to act, a friend was in trouble.

I hung up the phone, dreading the next wave of nausea I knew would come.

At the *Mesa Tribune,* Max Jennings hung up the telephone and yelled to the newsroom librarian.

"Sandy, get me the name of the head of the FDA in Washington."

As he talked, he was thumbing through his Rolodex for the private Washington number of Arizona Representative John Rhodes, the former House minority leader from Mesa. Representative Rhodes, beloved in Mesa and a veteran of thirty years in Congress, would help if he could. Max was sure of it. There was no answer at his Washington office. Max redialed and let the phone ring for a few times more before he remembered that it was President's Day, a federal holiday. He thumbed through his Rolodex, cursing to himself, and found Rhodes's home number in Washington. There was no answer.

Max slammed down the phone, his mind racing. He found the home number of an aide to Arizona Senator Barry Goldwater. Then, instead, he decided to try to find someone in the office of Arizona Senator Dennis DeConcini. Senator DeConcini had worked hard to get to know the people he represented. He had gathered a young, energetic staff that he had trained to be responsive. Max had dealt with some of Senator DeConcini's people before, and they possessed the kind of enthusiasm he needed now.

On a hunch he called DeConcini's Phoenix office. Despite the holiday, the phone was answered on the first ring.

Jennings was a veteran wire service reporter, foreign correspondent, and editor, and he had been hardened by his experiences. But they most often involved people he didn't know. He was wet eyed as he began to spill out his story to Mike Crusa, a young DeConcini aide. Jennings's voice was cracking as he summarized quickly the story for Crusa.

Crusa, too, seemed both touched by the story and outraged at the bureaucracy that was letting a woman needlessly die. He listened carefully and interrupted Max once or twice to get the spelling of the drug and the correct spelling of the names of my doctors. He was totally sympathetic.

"We've got to burn up those phone lines to Washington. Anything you can do will help," Max said. "I'm going to keep trying too."

"We'll help," Mike said. "But you know it's a holiday."

"I know that," Max said. "Mary can't wait any longer."

"I understand," Mike said. "We'll get back to you."

"Thanks," Max said. "I'll be here."

Max hung up and started dialing the number of an old friend from United Press International who worked in Washington. He had only begun his call when he looked at the clock and realized he had to call me back. He didn't have much to tell. He was disgusted with himself.

While Max was working, Karl and I sat quietly. "Max will do something," I told Karl. We had worked together on many projects and I felt he would respond to my call. I knew he understood my situation and realized how desperate I was.

When Max called me back, he was apologetic. He reminded me it was a federal holiday and that all Washington offices were closed. He told me he had placed a few phone calls and some people were helping. Max was silent for a minute, thinking, and then he told me he had called Senator DeConcini's office and talked to Mike Crusa. He related their conversation.

"I think he's going to help us, Mar," Max said. At work, he frequently dropped the "y" of my name. We were working together again, and he lapsed into the old habit. "We are doing our best," he said. "There may not be much we can do until the morning. Hang in there."

"I will," I promised dutifully, my voice so faint Max could hardly hear me. He stared at the wall after hanging up the phone, his mind racing. Sandy Johnson, the newspaper librarian, came running into his office.

"Max, here is the name of the head of the FDA you wanted."

He took the offered slip of paper and began to thumb his Rolodex again. As it turned out, he already had made the most important call in his quest.

At eight the next morning, Max called me.

"Mike Crusa, in DeConcini's office, is really working on this," Max said, speaking so loudly into the phone it was almost painful. "Mike talked to DeConcini. DeConcini is outraged by the holdup too. He is going to help!"

My spirits were lifted by Max's tone. I could tell he was feeling much better than he had the day before. I had a hunch he knew a lot more than he was telling me. He sounded optimistic.

An hour after we talked, the phone rang again. It was Bruce Reitz.

"Mary, who is Max Jennings?"

"Max Jennings is the executive editor of our paper. Why?"

"Well," Bruce asked, "how would you like to come to Stanford?"

"I'd love it. How about tomorrow? I don't think I can get myself together today." As I spoke I fought to keep down a rising hope. I didn't want another disappointment. "Why?"

"We've got the approval," Bruce said. Even his voice smiled. "It came in the last three hours. I can't believe it. I don't know what you did, but whatever it was, you didn't do it just for yourself. You did it for a lot of people. We've got blanket approval to use cyclosporin A for all heart-lung transplants."

I didn't have to hold the hope down any longer. I had literally received a new lease on life, at least from the perspective of someone who was as desperate as I was.

Bruce dismissed the politics of the situation quickly.

"I don't know what happened. Whatever it was, I'm not questioning it. When can you get out here?"

I answered quickly. "Tomorrow!"

I hung up the phone and dialed Karl's number.

"I'm going to Stanford tomorrow," I said.

"You're kidding!"

"No, I'm not." I quickly went over the phone calls of the morning. "I doubt even Max knows exactly what happened," I said. I was right. I never learned the answer to that question. All I knew was that through the efforts of Max and DeConcini, the Gordian knot of bureaucracy had been cut. I had a chance to live again.

At that moment, I was about as happy as I had ever been in my life. The day before, I was sure I would die at any moment. How suddenly I put that hurdle behind me and turned my attention to other things, to normal mundane details.

What clothes would I wear? I panicked. I remembered my favorite white blouse—the one I would have to take, of course—had a button missing and I had none to match it. I called my dear friend, Joyce Howland, and told her I was going to Stanford and that the transplant was on. Joyce let out a squeal and promised to come over immediately. She did, and she brought all new buttons for the blouse. Karl made it home in record time to find his normally quiet, somewhat forlorn home bustling with activity. He made Joyce a drink while she sewed on the buttons and chatted happily. Mother tried to keep things in perspective, to make sure I would not forget anything.

"Mary, are you packing underwear?" she demanded.

I laughed. "Mother, sit down and relax."

"Mary!" Mother scolded. "You don't have enough time to pack. We have got to get these things ready. We can't just sit around and talk."

I was not the slightest bit concerned. I was having a wonderful time, talking to Joyce, looking forward to something positive for a change. I can't explain how, at one moment, I could be so weak and forlorn and helpless and, the next, be laughing and plenty able to do things. The mind is always stronger than the body. I had something to do; I had a reason for going on.

As it turned out, Mother was right to ask questions. I went to Stanford without a slip.

Mother had to pack for herself too. We'd be at Stanford for months. Once there, I still had to wait, no one knew how long, for a donor. I couldn't wait alone, so Mother would be with me. Her commitment was just beginning. It would turn out to be an incredible one.

When Luke came home from school and found out what was happening, he was ebullient. He had always been sure luck would come my way. His happy excitement was contagious. The sun in his young face outshone the one in the Arizona sky.

Chris received the news without comment. I knew what he was thinking. He had never shared his brother's optimism. He was sure I would never return alive. He sat silent, holding his fear inside. He didn't want to hurt me, to rain on my parade.

The next day Karl, Mother, and I drove to the airport alone. One of the most difficult things I've ever done in my life was to leave the kids that morning. I wasn't worried about their physical care, I'd made arrangements for that long before. Luke would be staying with Haney and Joyce Womack who lived directly across our street. Chris, who was older and more responsible, would stay at home, but under the Womacks' watchful eyes. Karl would be coming back soon to stay with them until the donor organs were found. I would miss them so very much, but I knew I'd be back. If I hadn't been sure of that I don't think I could have left them. I had hugged them as hard as I could before we left and told them I loved them. I told them I'd be back and tried to reassure them, but mostly I told them I loved them. I had to be sure they knew that no matter what happened.

The only people to see us off were Max Jennings and the head photographer from the *Mesa Tribune,* Don Stevenson. I was glad to see Max. We had never been social friends, but I was comforted that he came to see me off. Max was a link with a profession I enjoyed, a happy part of my life, and one I hoped to return to. He was a reminder that I had a future.

I was wheeled to the door of the plane in a wheelchair and stood up shakily. I turned to Max, gave him a hug, stepped back, and smiled weakly.

I was using my last reserves, and I think Max knew it. He was wet eyed. He, like most of my friends, was sure he'd never see me again. It would take long to convince him of what I knew. He was wrong. I'd be back. I was going to live.

NINE

San Jose was beautiful. I sat in a wheelchair by the door to the terminal and admired the bright sunshine while Karl collected the luggage and rented a car. I would have thought it beautiful if it had been raining and cold. I was in San Jose, barely twenty miles from Stanford. I had a chance to live, a real chance.

Mother was talking to me, but I paid no attention. I was too preoccupied with my own thoughts, my own joy.

Karl came with the car and the two of us piled in. As usual, I admonished Karl to drive slowly (I'm a terrible backseat driver). But this time I really didn't mean it. I was in a hurry to get there.

I wasn't the only one in a rush. When I checked into the hospital, a waiting army of technicians immediately launched a series of tests—blood tests, tissue tests, more blood tests, X rays, eye tests. Sometimes I think hospitals keep a few vampires on staff. I don't know what else they do with all the blood.

Mother stayed with me. Karl, after I was checked in, left to find a motel and unload the baggage from the car. I was anxious to see Bruce Reitz again. Although I had often talked to him, I hadn't seen him since October. He promised he would stop in to visit me. It was to be the first of many promises, and he would keep them all.

They finally finished the tests for the day. There would be more tomorrow. I lay back on the bed and was resting when Bruce stuck his head in the door. When he saw I was awake, he walked over and took my hand gently in his own.

"You're here," he said.

"You bet I am." I smiled at him. "And I'm ready."

Bruce did not reply at first. He held my hand for a long time, then said softly, "I'm so glad to see you."

I kept smiling to fight back the tears. I couldn't speak for a moment.

"I don't know what you did," Bruce said. "I never saw anything move so fast."

I grinned at him. "Well, Bruce, I told you I was a street fighter. I just got tired of all the waiting and of all the bullshit and decided if I wasn't going to make it, it wasn't going to be my fault."

"Well," he replied quickly, "you're going to make it. You did it."

"I did it with help," I said.

He asked what had happened.

He sat and listened intently. As I told him about calling Max Jennings at the newspaper, he grinned. When I went through the details, ending with my trip to California, his grin broadened.

"You gotta learn to be a fighter," I lectured him. "You gotta remember this for everyone else."

Bruce's grin broke into a laugh. "I think I'm going to have to hire you as my assistant to get things done, after the surgery that is."

Bruce left, promising to return with the other members of the transplant team.

My euphoria, if anything, increased. I felt at that moment as if I was beginning the greatest adventure of my life and that I would survive. For the first time in months, I felt really secure. If something happened, I would be taken care of. For months I had been aware that my life was threatened, that I could die any day. At home I had secretly worried that if something happened to me there, I had no option but to die. Now, I felt like a child with a security blanket.

"Safe," I thought. "That's what it is, I feel safe."

Part of my comfort came from the nursing staff on that first day. They bustled in and out of the room to check on me, to take tests, and sometimes just to visit. I felt as if my hospital room had come with a built-in cheerleading section. The nurses were excited and they made no effort to hide it. I decided the nurses really liked working at Stanford Hospital. They had their own form of patriotism. They cared about this hospital, and they cared about me.

The sun was setting. I couldn't see it, but I still thought it was a beautiful sunset. I was resting when Bruce returned, accompanied by two other doctors, Dr. John Wallwork, an English surgeon from Cambridge who was studying transplant techniques, and Dr. John Pennock, a member of the transplant team. They would be intimately associated with my case, and Bruce wanted me to get to know them.

I immediately liked Dr. Wallwork, a pudgy, jovial man with wild blond hair who told me, "We're the ones you're going to hate sometimes."

I laughed. "Why am I going to hate you?"

"Don't worry," he promised, a cheerful smile bisecting his round face. "You will, but we want an honest and open relationship. Down the road there will be times when you will hate us all. Let it out. Tell us about it. It's going to be a long, hard road. You'll get mad at us and we'll get mad at you. It won't be fun and games but we must work together."

I was sure now I liked John Wallwork. He was up front and direct. I told him, "You don't know me yet. You'll find out that if I have something to say, you'll hear it."

All three doctors sobered as Bruce said, "There must be many things about the surgery you want to know. We'll try to always keep you informed of everything, but any questions you have, ask any of us."

I nodded. "To be frank, it isn't the surgery itself I'm interested in. I probably couldn't understand it anyway. I don't know anything about medicine. What interests me is what happens afterward?"

"For the first twenty-four hours, you'll be on a ventilator to help you breathe," Bruce said. "Don't try to talk when you are on the ventilator. You won't be able to speak anyway, but if you try, you'll have a very sore throat afterward because there will be a tube down your throat.

"The first critical moment comes when we remove the ventilator and you have to breathe on your own.

"The next critical point is the healing of your trachea, your windpipe, where your new lungs will be attached. The steroids you have to take to prevent rejection also interfere with healing, and the trachea is slow to heal anyway. By using cyclosporin we can reduce the amount of steroids and healing should proceed well. It has in the monkeys."

Bruce's descriptions didn't sound exactly cheerful, but I wasn't surprised by what he said. I knew the risk and I was prepared to take it. I felt a tension building inside me and wanted to break it.

"How's the monkey doing anyway?" I asked.

"You mean Momma?" John Wallwork said. "She's doing fine."

"Well, see that you take care of her," I told him.

Bruce continued his description. "Apart from those two problems I mentioned, your recovery will be similar to that of a heart transplant patient. We have to be careful of infections. After the first week or so they are the biggest danger."

Bruce went on quietly telling me of the many things that could happen. I'd probably go into rejection. My body would try to fight off the new organs as if they were an invader, but the doctors knew how to handle that. There were no guarantees. Hell, there never are. I could recover, walk out of the hospital, and be run over by a truck. All they, and I, could do was to try our damnedest. I was sure they would and I knew I was going to. No guarantee, but more important, I had a real chance.

We were all quiet for a few minutes while I digested what I had been told. Finally I asked one more question, one that had been bothering me, nagging at the back of my mind, for some time.

"What about the donor?"

"We've already started looking for the donor. We never know how long that will take."

"I don't mean that," I interrupted. I was suddenly dealing with the reality that for me to live, someone else had to die.

"I know what you mean, Mary," Bruce said. "Just remember, whoever your donor is, that person would have died anyway, even if no transplant were ever performed. You shouldn't feel guilty. You are in no way responsible.

"Your feelings aren't unusual. That is one of the reasons we never tell transplant patients the names of their donors. It's better on both sides. Sometimes when the families of donors learn the name of the recipient it causes psychological problems for them. They begin to believe their loved one isn't really dead, that he or she still lives inside the body of a total stranger."

We talked a little more, and then the three doctors left. Bruce was right about the donor. Intellectually I understood that any transplant depended on someone's death, but I still harbored a little nagging feeling of guilt that I would profit from so tragic an event. I guess I always will.

The next day Karl began apartment hunting, working from a list provided him by Lois Christopherson. He found a place within walking distance of the medical center. The woman who owned it was not sure she wanted to rent to us because she had rental guaranteed for the following summer. Karl liked the apartment and thought I would too, but he hadn't been able to close the deal. When he told me about the holdup, I called the apartment owner, Linda Austin, to try to get her to change her mind. It was just another sales call.

"We really need this apartment," I told Linda. "I'm going to the hospital soon. I really hope you will give us first consideration."

I had no idea how long we would need the apartment, and this turned out to be the sticking point. After a while, I called Linda again.

This time she yielded. "Phooey, I'm not going to worry about next summer. I'm not sure I can let you have it after June, because I did promise to rent it to someone then. We can worry about that in June."

Karl met Linda Austin and rented the apartment, then came over to the hospital to tell me everything was settled. I had a place to live.

"How much is it?" I had not asked before.

"Seven fifty a month," he said.

"My God!" I was shocked. "For a one bedroom. How are we going to afford it?"

"Don't worry, honey," he answered, calm as usual. "Believe me, it's a damned good price for this area and we'll find a way to survive. Just take it easy on expenses—nothing that isn't necessary. I'll take care of the rest."

I had doubts, but I took Karl's word that everything would be all right. We had used our savings and taken a second mortgage on the house to clean up all our bills. I knew some of that money was left, and if Karl said it was okay, it was.

I did not find out until long afterward how tight things really were. Our living expenses skyrocketed with two homes to support. Karl and the boys went on a Spartan diet, no snacks and sodas. They stayed home. The boys' spending money was limited to what they could earn on their own. Karl borrowed what money he could, but he told no one the true state of our finances, not even me. He felt all I could do about it was worry. He was right.

Mother and Karl moved in immediately. I remained in the hospital five days before the tests were completed. The fourth-floor suite was modern and cheerful. There was a balcony with a huge window. Rolling green hills leading up to the edge of the Stanford campus made a beautiful view. I loved it. It was a happy place, yet quiet and peaceful. I was content there. I hoped to be going home by June. I didn't dream we would be there for seven months.

Karl left on Monday to go back to work. He had to; our creditors were sympathetic about my problems—as long as the bills were paid on time. He was prepared to return within minutes of a phone call.

There was little for Mother and me to do while we waited for the donor. I had orders to call the hospital every half hour when I went somewhere, a constant reminder that the call could come at any moment. The restrictions didn't bother me much; I didn't have the strength to go sightseeing.

I was fearful about the beautiful plants in the apartment. Every plant I had ever tried to raise had died. Mother promised she would take care of them. Like everything under Mother's loving care, the plants prospered.

Occasionally the two of us went window-shopping. I recalled Karl's gentle reminders that we didn't have a lot of excess cash. Mother and I didn't need lots of money. We had wonderful lunches together and long talks. We began to know each other again. We had both changed in the twenty-eight years since I had left home. We would become much, much closer in the months ahead.

On the morning of March 4, I received my official San Francisco Bay welcome. I was sleeping on the sofa bed in the living room and Mother was on the water bed in the bedroom when the apartment began to sway. Mother came running out of the bedroom and the two of us sat petrified while the apartment building rocked. I could see my epitaph: "Killed by an earthquake while awaiting a transplant."

The next day, as I was being examined by Dr. Reitz, I asked him, "Bruce, did you feel the earthquake last night?"

He looked at me, mildly surprised. "No, was there one?"

The earthquake had put a question in my mind.

"Bruce," I asked, "do you have all this information stored away somewhere, on microfilm? At the Library of Congress? What if an earthquake were to destroy the university?"

He grinned. "It's just here," he said. "If it all goes, we all go. What does it matter?"

"Hell, it matters if people elsewhere could interpret your work," I responded quickly. I was troubled by the conversation and didn't share Dr. Reitz's sense of humor. I still worry what would happen if all the transplant files and information were destroyed.

Mother perpetually tried to make me eat while I awaited the transplant. She cooked my favorite dishes every day. But for the most part, I just picked at the food. I weighed about ninety pounds, ten pounds fewer than normal. I was more aware than anyone else that my strength was failing.

I had a lot of time to think, and my mind kept returning to thoughts about the organs I needed. For the second time in my life, someone else's loss would be my gain. The first time was when we adopted our children. That was one of my very happiest moments. Now, my life itself depended on someone else. I still felt a deep sadness at the thought that my survival depended on the death of another. It bothered me, but I told myself as I waited, "I can live with that." Gradually as the days leading up to the surgery went by, I began to feel better. I couldn't explain why, except that my confidence began to grow. I felt I would have the operation and I would survive.

Karl and I talked most days by phone. Ma Bell was getting richer, if no one else. There was seldom any news. It was good just to talk to each other.

Karl was waiting to hear any moment that a donor had been found. He was busy at work and he was thankful for that. Karl is an electronics engineer and was designing some kind of satellite communications equipment. He possesses a great ability to concentrate on a problem, and this ability helped to take his mind temporarily off what was ahead for all of us. Like me, he was anxious. He knew the wait could last months. He knew better than anyone else that I could slip away from him forever during one of my blackouts.

March 8 came, a Sunday. Mother and I worked our way through the bulky San Jose Sunday paper. It was a warm spring afternoon and the door to the balcony was open. Mother had splurged for a change and we were having crab legs for dinner. We were discussing what we were going to have with our treat. The telephone rang.

It was 1:30 P.M. I picked up the phone and recognized Bruce Reitz's voice.

"Mary?"

"Hi, Bruce."

He called frequently, so I was not alarmed.

"What's up?" I asked.

"Mary, I'd like to have you at the hospital in the next thirty or forty minutes. I believe we have a donor."

"Oh?" was all I could say. For a moment I had absolutely nothing to say. My mind went blank. The moment I had awaited so long had arrived, and I didn't know what to say. I sat staring into the phone.

I think Mother knew instantly. All she could do was mumble dumbly, "What is it?"

"They have a donor."

Mother got up and left the room for a moment while I continued to talk to Bruce.

"Okay, thirty minutes?" I asked him again, my mind barely functioning.

"Yes."

"Okay. I'll have to call Karl."

"I'll see you in a half hour."

"But Bruce, we were going to have crab legs for dinner tonight. I guess I can't eat, right?"

I smiled into the phone. It was the biggest moment of my life and nothing but stupid inconsequential things entered my mind.

The voice on the other end of the phone was gentle. "No, Mary, I would prefer you didn't." I knew he was smiling too.

As I hung up the phone, Mother came back into the room. She walked over and put her arms around me.

"What do we take to the hospital?"

"Hell, I don't know," I said. We both knew it would be a long, long time before I needed anything the hospital wouldn't provide.

I called Karl. When I heard his voice, I started to cry. He knew instantly why I had called.

"Karl, you must come out," I said. "I want to talk to the boys."

Chris was the first on the phone.

"Chris, they have the donor and I'm going into surgery at about six o'clock," I began. He didn't say anything. I continued. "Chris, I want you to know how much I love you and how much I care about you, and no matter what happens, the important thing is that you try. It doesn't matter if you don't always win. It matters that you tried. I want you to always remember that. I love you." I only realized that moment that I had been thinking about the speech for a long time.

Chris was silent for a moment. "Okay, Mom. I love you."

I told Luke the same thing in different words.

"You know, Luke, think of it this way: not everybody gets A's in school. But you try to do the best you can do. That's what I did, and I want you to remember." Then I switched into another tense.

"I'll see you whenever you come up."

"You're going to make it, Mother. Don't worry," Luke said. "I'll be up to see you."

When Karl got back on the phone, neither of us could speak for a minute. I sobbed. I was afraid I'd go to surgery without seeing him again. Seeing Karl again became terribly important.

"Honey, I'll be there," he promised. "I've got to go now because I have a plane to catch."

Mother threw a few things into a bag while I called a cab. As she closed the door to the apartment and we started down the hall, I wondered what was ahead of me. If I'd known then, I'd still have gone.

TEN

At fifteen minutes past six, Karl burst through the door of my room at Stanford Medical Center. I smiled. I needed him and I needed to know he was there. I'd been worried I'd go to surgery before he arrived. Karl gave me a kiss and then stood at my bedside for a few moments.

"Well, honey," he finally said. "I made it. I was worried I wouldn't make it before you went to surgery. How is everything going?"

"All right, I guess," I answered. "There is some kind of holdup with the donor. I really don't know what it is."

Karl's brow furrowed, but he said nothing. The same idea was in both our minds—the possibility of a false alarm. We had been warned that sometimes, for a variety of reasons, a transplant candidate is called and then sent home again. Despite the warning, we didn't want to face that possibility. Maybe I'd have to go home again and wait for another donor. Maybe Karl had come 800 miles for nothing. I didn't care about that part, I was glad to see him again.

I had already passed one hurdle before Karl arrived. I had been thoroughly examined again. The doctors had to be sure I had no low-grade infection of any kind. Donor or no donor, I couldn't have a transplant if I had any infection.

Earlier, when I checked into the hospital, Mother and I were taken to a small room where three other patients were being prepared for surgery. It was the last time I would share a hospital room. Transplant recipients must have private rooms. The immunosuppressant drugs we must take for the rest of our lives leave us too subject to infection to take the chance of sharing hospital rooms. I listened to one woman who was going to have a gallbladder operation. She was petrified and confided her fears to the other patients. I smiled and said to Mother, "I should be so lucky."

Larry, a male nurse whom I had met earlier, popped in and out several times as I waited. He kept reassuring me that everything was going to be all right. There was often delay in a transplant. The staff always wanted to be sure the recipient was there early. Larry was both a comfort and a help. He helped me shuffle through the stack of forms I had to sign. Because the transplant operation was experimental, there were more forms than for the usual operation. I read them. There was nothing in them I hadn't expected, but one of them would haunt me in an odd way a couple of weeks later.

We finally finished, and Larry sat down on the edge of the bed and took my hand. "What are you thinking about?" he asked.

I was startled at the question because it made me realize I was doing exactly that—thinking—thinking back over my life, about my children, my husband, my relatives and friends. I was mentally taking stock. It would have taken hours to answer Larry's question. I just smiled and shook my head. Karl, my mother, and I sat and made small talk. We couldn't discuss what was on all of our minds. I was going to have a heart-lung transplant. We knew that, but what did it really mean? What was ahead? How was it going to affect our lives? We all had the same questions. But what were the answers?

Bruce Reitz came in to see me several times. He only stopped a few minutes each visit. I could tell he was agitated by the delay. There was nothing he could do for me until the donor arrived. I think he wanted to get started. I knew I did.

Dr. Mark Heilberman, who was to be my anesthesiologist, came to see me. He stood at the foot of my bed and talked to the three of us for a long time, explaining what would be happening in the operating room.

"After the operation, you won't be taken to the recovery room as a normal surgery patient would."

I had already known that, but his next words surprised me.

"We'll bring you back to consciousness again while you are still in the operating room. Just long enough to see that you are going to come out of the anesthetic. We'll then put you back out. You'll be taken directly to your room and put on a ventilator.

"You won't feel a great deal of pain. In fact, you'll never remember the first day or two after the operation."

He was wrong there. I remember virtually nothing of the first three weeks after the operation.

The telephone rang. It was for Dr. Heilberman. After he hung up the phone, he came over to my bed again.

"I'll be going now, Mary. I have to get ready. They are bringing the donor in. See you later."

Larry entered a few minutes after Dr. Heilberman left and told me they would be coming for me soon. I looked at Mother and Karl. They looked back. None of us knew what to say. Mother put her arms around me and kissed me.

"I love you" were her only words. Her eyes were filled with tears.

Karl put his arms around me and held me for a long

minute. "I love you, honey, and don't worry. Everything is going to be all right."

"Karl, if anything happens, I mean, if I don't make it . . . I don't have to tell you to take care of the kids, I know you will, but once in a while put your arms around them and tell them you love them. They need that."

Karl nodded, then backed away from the bed. A man with a gurney was there to take me to the operating room. He helped me climb on. Karl and Mother walked beside me as I was slowly wheeled through the hospital corridors to the double doors at the entrance to the operating rooms. When we reached the entrance, we stopped and they each kissed me again. Karl said, "I'll see you in the morning, Mary."

I suppose I should have had something profound to say as I entered, but I couldn't think of it. All I said was, "Well, this is it."

The pneumatic doors hissed a greeting as I was rolled through. The corridor leading to the operating rooms was bland and austere. Jim, the attendant who wheeled me in, stopped at the operating room door. He couldn't take me in because he wasn't sterile. From this moment forward I would live in a sterile environment for several months.

I had never seen an operating room before, not while I was fully conscious that is. In the middle of the room was the operating table. I wondered how I'd fit on it. It looked too narrow to hold even me and I was only five feet and weighed barely a hundred pounds. They lifted me onto the table and I looked around. Strangely I wasn't nervous or afraid. There were about a dozen people in the room, but I couldn't recognize a soul. They were all masked and gowned for the operation. Green forms with eyes was all I could see.

"Is Dr. Reitz here?" I asked no one in particular, just the green-gowned group.

"I'm here, Mary." His gentle voice was unmistakable. He came over and took my hand, but didn't say more. I think he was impatient with the delays. Looking past my feet, I could see a clock on the far wall. It was ten o'clock.

Dr. Heilberman was behind my head and I couldn't see him. He kept talking to me, explaining anything I wanted to know. I think he wanted to comfort me and be sure I wasn't getting too apprehensive.

The operating room was rather large with a surprisingly low ceiling, about the height of an average room. I don't know why, but I had expected it to be higher. Overhead were the lights they would use during the operation. They were off now. There were boxes piled along the walls. Mark Heilberman told me they contained things that probably wouldn't be used in this operation. They were there because they might be needed. Anything they could conceivably need was already in the room.

To my left a nurse was laying out the instruments at a long table. It must have been more than six feet in length. I could hear the soft murmur of her voice as she counted each one.

"Make sure you count the same number when you're done," I told her. She laughed.

"I will."

Two weeks later I received a card from the operating room nurses. The card said, "I counted!"

All around the room people stood in little groups. I could hear the mingled sound of their voices as they talked, but none loudly enough to make out what they were talking about. Bruce Reitz wasn't conversing with anyone. He paced back and forth at the far end of the room. He was going to try something that had never successfully been done before. He, and I, were about to step over a threshold. I respected his aloneness.

To my left was a huge metal box. Dr. Heilberman told me it was the heart-lung machine. They would open it later.

The people in the room kept milling around, forming and reforming into little groups. I guess they were all getting a little impatient. Some of the masked figures were doctors, some were nurses and technicians. One was a photographer who would take pictures for the hospital records. Dr. Norman Shumway, originator of the transplant program at Stanford, was present. He would assist in the operation. Some of the doctors were there to assist, some to observe, some to learn. I didn't know who was who.

I finally recognized John Wallwork. His bright, merry, blue eyes peering between the mask and cap were unmistakable. I didn't know it at the moment, of course, but Wallwork had had an exhausting day of his own. That morning, the hospital donor alert system had contacted Stanford with the news that a teenager in suburban San Diego had suffered a bicycle accident and was a possible donor. John immediately flew down to San Diego to run tests on the brain-dead body. Once it was established that the heart and lungs were satisfactory, John flew back to Stanford with the donor, who was kept alive until the time of surgery. This is standard procedure in heart-lung transplants, because the donor organs cannot be preserved outside the body for very long. A heart can be removed from the donor and kept in a saline solution, but the heart and lungs together cannot. Wallwork's job also included removing the organs from the donor's body and preparing them to be transplanted.

I had my hand around the IV stand alongside the operating table. Suddenly the stand began to shake. It was my hand shaking it; my whole body was trembling uncontrollably.

"Bruce, I'd like to put her out now," Dr. Heilberman said. "Is it all right?"

"Yes," Bruce answered. "You had better put her under now."

I looked at the clock. It showed 12:15 A.M. I wouldn't have my transplant on Sunday after all. It was Monday, March 9, 1981.

ELEVEN

MOTHER AND KARL WATCHED AS I WAS TAKEN THROUGH THE doors to the operating rooms. The doors closed, and they stood there unsure of what to do or where to go. A nurse took them to the waiting room near the North Intensive Care Unit, more commonly called NICU. They would wait there through the night. Fortunately, they didn't have to wonder what was going on while they waited. The nurses on NICU kept them informed about what was happening. There was really little to hear. For the first two hours they waited just as I did. Once the operation started, no word was expected until forty-five minutes before I was ready to be brought from the operating room. The forty-five-minute warning was for the nurses. My room had to be ready.

Actually the preparation of my room started even before Bruce began to operate. Soon after Mother and Karl arrived at NICU, Barbara, the charge nurse on NICU, showed them my room. It was one of five special rooms used for the care of transplant patients. Called reverse isolation rooms, they were designed to protect the patient from exposure to infection. My immune system was completely suppressed to discourage rejection of the donor organs. One of the most serious concerns of my doctors was that I would get an infection. Even a minor infection could be fatal because my body had no way to fight it.

The reverse isolation room was really a double room, consisting of an inner room and a small anteroom where anyone entering would put on a sterile gown and mask. When Mother and Karl first saw it, the inner room was bare; everything had been taken out to allow it to be scrubbed and sterilized. Someone was already at work. The inner room was only slightly larger than the usual private hospital room, and by the time all of the equipment was moved back in, it seemed smaller. There were monitors to keep a check on my new heart and respiration rate and a ventilator to help me breathe during the first twenty-four hours after the operation. There was a lot of other equipment as well, some of which the physical therapists would use to help me regain my strength and to exercise my new lungs. Several machines were for emergencies. The defibrillator would be used only if my heartbeat became erratic, and the paddles would be used to shock my heart in case it stopped. Some of the equipment in my room remained a mystery to me. Actually, I didn't really want to know what it was for. Much of it was clustered around the head of my bed, with the monitoring equipment to my right and behind me. The larger units were to my left, with the defibrillator on a shelf five feet from the floor. There was even a telephone, which usually stayed on top of the defibrillator and out of the way. It would be weeks before I would take any interest in the phone. Near the window was a desk the nurse used while updating my records, and where I could sit and write if I wished. Finally, at the other end, stood a cupboard, sink, and several shelves. The cupboard and shelves were stocked with enough drugs and medical supplies to fill a small pharmacy. Long before the operation was finished, my room was ready, everything in it but a bed. The bed had been taken to the operating room. When the operation was completed, I'd be brought, bed and all, straight from the operating room to this room in which I would spend the next few months.

Neither Karl nor my mother had eaten since noon. The hospital cafeteria was already closed by the time I was taken to the operating room. I told them to go out and have a good dinner when I went in for the operation. They didn't go; neither of them was about to leave the hospital. I guess I would have felt the same way. There is a snack bar in the basement, and they went down to get a sandwich from the machines. I don't think either of them had much of an appetite.

When Mother and Karl returned to the NICU waiting room, there was a surprise waiting for them: they couldn't get in. Uniformed guards were all over the place. No one was allowed into the NICU area unless he or she had business there. Stanford knew what we had been warned of—the media would get on the story as soon as it broke, and it had already broken. The people at Stanford don't mind making history, but they prefer to do it quietly. Most of all, they are concerned about the patient. I would not be able to stand the attention. For the next few months, I would have all I could do to stay alive, and they were going to be damned sure nothing interfered with my recovery. I must say that my experience with the media was good. They wanted the story, but they tried to respect my privacy and for the most part did an excellent job.

One of the nurses came out and identified my mother and Karl to the guards. The head of the security unit took them around to meet all the guards. After that they had no trouble getting in and out. I can't say the same for the nurses that night. Even my primary nurse, Audrey Covner, had to show her hospital identification badge to get into the unit. But she had left it at home—most nights there was no need for identification, everyone on the unit knew her. This night, when she reported, she had to turn around, go home, get her ID, and return. She wasn't the only one.

Karl and Mother settled down for the long wait that night. Barbara came out and asked if they wanted pillows and a blanket so they could rest. Neither of them did. Sleep was out of the question. Karl found the nurses' coffee pot, helped himself, settled down, and tried to read. He read little that night. Mother quietly worried. Karl tried to comfort her, but there was little he could say—he was worried himself.

Finally about 4:30 A.M. Audrey came out and told Karl and Mother the operation was finished, they were closing, and I would be out in about forty-five minutes. It was the best news they had received all night. Still they had to wait. If the wait had already seemed long, it was interminable now. Finally Dr. Reitz and Dr. Wallwork came out to see them. Both were happy. The operation had gone well. The donor organs were healthy and had been an excellent fit. My new heart had started spontaneously and was beating well. There had been no surprises.

Bruce told Karl and my mother that I would be out in about fifteen minutes, but it would be an hour before they could see me. Karl wanted to know why. He was uncharacteristically impatient. Bruce explained that I had to be prepared, the ventilator attached to help me breathe, tubes attached to drain my chest, and several other complicated procedures performed.

Mother and Karl walked down the hall to the operating room exit to see me as I came by. They didn't get a very long look. The doors burst open and three attendants brought me through, one holding the IV bottles elevated and the other two guiding the bed. They weren't running, it just seemed that way. I was hardly a candidate for a beauty contest. I suppose I looked as if I had been through a war and lost. In a matter of a few seconds I was gone—taken to my room.

After the predicted hour, Karl and Mother were led there also. A nurse showed Mother and Karl how to put on the gowns, hats, and booties. Mother needed help with the booties; she was still having trouble with the knee she had broken before coming to Arizona. Finally they put on gloves and masks and could enter the inner room.

Karl and Mother came into my room and over to my bed. I was still asleep. Karl didn't know what to do. He wanted to talk to me, to let me know he was there, but he was afraid I would try to answer him and he had been told I shouldn't try to talk as long as the ventilator was in. Bruce Reitz told Karl and Mother it was all right for them to speak to me, but not to expect any response. I was still pretty heavily doped up.

Karl spoke. "I'm here Mary," he said. "Don't try to talk, you just rest. Everything is going to be all right."

I was covered by a sheet up to the top of my chest, but Karl could see the top of my incision. He was surprised. It showed only as a fine line, and there were no visible stitches. He asked Bruce about it.

"You just can't see the stitches," Bruce told him. "The breastbone is held together by metal clamps and the suturing is under the skin. That part of the operation is just like any open-heart surgery."

Karl nodded and came back over to stand beside me. He put his hand on my arm, and even through the gloves he could feel how cold I was. During the operation my body had been cooled to seventy-seven degrees, and it would be about twenty-four hours before I would warm up again. That was one of the reasons I was kept sedated for the first day. If I woke up, I would be freezing.

I know that Karl and Mother were present only because they have told me about it. I can remember nothing of those early days after my transplant. Oddly enough, I do remember waking up in the operating room as Mark Heilberman had foretold. I heard him say, "Should I give her more oxygen, Bruce, or anesthetic?"

"Oxygen," I heard Bruce answer. "Give her oxygen."

Bruce explained to Karl and Mother what they were doing to stabilize me. I was being given blood, not a lot; amazingly, I had lost relatively little during the operation. He warned them I would soon turn yellow, jaundiced, because the heart-lung machine, which had kept me alive for over two hours while the transplant was performed, had crushed some of my blood cells. All my internal organs had nearly stopped functioning as a result of my body's being cooled during the operation. It would be a few days before my liver worked well enough to clean the dead cells out of my blood.

Karl, ever the cautious scientist, checked my blood transfusion to be sure it was type O. He noticed that some of the blood being used was Rh positive and some was negative. He asked Bruce about it.

Bruce told him gently that the Rh factor wasn't important in transfusions. If he ever tired of answering Karl's questions, he never showed it. Over the next few weeks Karl wanted to know everything that was happening. Karl can handle worries better if he knows what's going on. Having a grip on the facts makes him more comfortable. Mother, on the other hand, remained relatively uninterested in the medical details of the operation, and throughout she preferred to deal with me on an instinctive level, the way she had always done.

Each time I was given blood that first day, one nurse would read the patient number and the blood type required and another nurse would read from the blood supply the patient number for whom the blood was intended and the blood type. The ritual comforted Karl. The nurses were constantly busy, monitoring heart rate and blood pressure, taking samples for analyses of blood gases and chemical factors, giving medication, and heaven knows what else. In short, the nurses worked to keep me alive. If I didn't make it, it wasn't going to be because of a lack of effort on their part.

About three hours after I was brought from the operating room, Karl left my room and got a cup of coffee. He also had a job to do. He had promised me he would keep my newspaper, and only my newspaper, informed. He really wasn't interested in talking to the media. To be truthful, he really didn't think most of the media would be interested either. Also he had another motive. Karl wanted to ask Haney Womack to let Luke know that everything had gone all right. Luke was in school, and although it was doubtful that he would learn anything that day, this little bit of news would keep him content. Haney would answer his questions until Karl could call Luke that evening.

After Karl talked to Haney, he called Max Jennings and answered a barrage of questions as well as he could. Unknown to Karl, Max had become the unofficial press spokesman for the family. Max was besieged with calls from everywhere, as was the public information office at Stanford Medical Center. Karl had been wrong. The media were interested. Regardless of the interest, he could tell Max little other than the news that the operation had gone as planned.

Karl ate breakfast and came back to my room to find Mother hovering by the side of my bed as if something would happen if she took her eyes off me for a moment Never would the doctors discourage Mother from her vigil. They wanted the family there; they always felt that family support was an important part of the recovery process.

The day went by, Mother hovering, the doctors and nurses working, and Karl keeping watch. I, for my part, was oblivious to it all. Between the trauma of the operation and the drugs I was on, my mind had retreated to the sole function of keeping my body working. I guess that was enough.

I only have one recollection of the first day, other than the brief moment of consciousness in the operating room.

About 10 P.M., Chris arrived. He was exhausted. He had driven Karl's car up from Mesa so Karl would have a car during my stay. Tired or not, the first thing he wanted to do was to see me.

Karl took him into the antechamber and initiated him into the process of dressing to visit a transplant patient. Karl was becoming an expert already. As he helped Chris on with the gown, he could feel him trembling. He put his arm around Chris's shoulder.

"Don't be worried Chris." He tried to reassure him. "Mother is doing fine. I don't need to tell you that Mother has been through a lot. Just don't expect too much. She can't talk and is pretty heavily sedated. She probably won't recognize you."

Karl was wrong there. First I heard a voice. It was Mother's voice, but it seemed to come from far away. I could hear her saying, "Mary, Mary, Chris is here."

I turned my head a little to the left, toward the door. I had no trouble recognizing the green-clad form. The frightened eyes peering at me could belong to only one person, my son Chris.

"It's Chris, Mary," Mother said again. "Say something to her, Chris. Go ahead. You can talk to her. She can't talk to you, but you can talk to her."

Chris reached out his big hand and gently touched my arm.

"How are you?"

"Poor kid," I thought. Even in my foggy mind, I sympathized with him. He didn't know what to say. Who would? I wanted to comfort him. I guess I must have remembered the admonition not to try to talk; anyway, I didn't. My hand was shaking badly, but I managed to raise it a few inches. I tried to put my thumb and forefinger together. I didn't succeed too well, but they all caught my meaning, I was OK.

I tried to smile at Chris. My lips were taped to the ventilator tube and I doubt they moved an eighth of an inch. It was enough; they all saw. I don't remember any more of Chris's first visit.

He didn't stay long. He was close to exhaustion and Karl knew it. On top of that, seeing me must have been a terrible strain. After about ten minutes, I had fallen asleep. Karl took Mother by the arm, and the three of them returned to the apartment. Chris wasn't the only one who was tired; both Mother and Karl had been up for over thirty hours.

They all plunged into bed immediately. I doubt an earthquake would have awakened them that night. Still, by six in the morning, Karl was back at the hospital. He found me looking exactly the same as when he had left. I didn't appear to have moved. Audrey was on duty. She told Karl that I was stable and all my vital signs were good. Bruce Reitz walked into the room. Karl thought he looked remarkably fresh and cheerful. Karl knew, from talking to the nurses, that Bruce hadn't gone home. Maybe he caught a nap at the hospital, but I don't know how. I wasn't his only patient.

About 9:30 A.M., Bruce, John Wallwork, and John Pennock, together with three nurses, came into my room. It was time to take me off the ventilator and see if I could breathe on my own. Karl left the room. There were six people in there to take care of me already and it was a small room. He knew he would only be in the way.

It was a critical moment and they all knew it. The nerves to my diaphragm had been removed and reattached during the operation, and there was a possibility they wouldn't function. A few minutes later Bruce emerged from my room to see Karl. I was breathing on my own. My new lungs had enough volume to sustain me.

They removed the tube from my throat before Karl returned. He met John Wallwork on the way into the room. John looked as if he had been given a present. Karl sat down beside my bed and held my hand a little while. Finally, I opened my eyes and looked at him.

"Karl. Karl, I made it," I said.

"Yes, honey, you sure did," Karl spoke softly. "You're doing pretty good. Don't worry about anything. Don't try to talk to me. You need your rest."

Karl stayed with me for a short while longer, then left for the apartment to get Mother and Chris. It was raining when he reached the parking lot. He thought it was a beautiful day.

TWELVE

Our lives had been torn up and transplanted just as had my heart and lungs. Like most people, we adapted quickly and fell into a new set of routines. For my part, lethargy dominated my life. I couldn't seem to get up either the energy or the will to do anything but lie in bed. My nurses would have no part of that—I had to get up for part of the day at least, even if only to sit in the chair.

Mother and Karl spent most of their time at the hospital, often just sitting while I slept. There was little for them to do, but Mother particularly felt a compulsion to be there. They tried to talk to me, to get me interested again in the world around me, but I wasn't cooperating. I think it was partly because of the drugs I was on and the aftereffects of the operation. I really didn't sleep very much. I was restless, constantly asking Mother or Karl to fix my pillow or to rub my back. I imagine I must have driven them half-crazy, but they never complained, just fixed my pillow or rubbed my back.

Mail began to arrive: cards and letters from all over the world, messages of hope and cheer, congratulations from people I had never met. The mail continued to come all the time I was in the hospital. It is still coming.

Mother read and reread each piece of mail. She would read it to me and show me the cards. At best, my response was a grunt. In those first days I couldn't seem to arouse any interest.

Karl tried to read novels, but they couldn't keep his attention. Instead, he read my charts and medical records. They were always in my room. He read articles on transplant surgery dating back fifteen years. He read the doctor's description of my operation. He read the pathology report. The report confirmed what the doctors had told us: the transplant had not come a moment too soon. My lungs were purplish and dying because of the inadequate blood supply. My heart was extremely enlarged on the right side and the muscle was paper thin. If the donor organs had arrived a few weeks later, I wouldn't have been there for the transplant. It was a near thing.

Karl found macabre humor in the description of the operation itself. It was written in precise, highly technical language describing each step of the operation, what was cut, how the organs were removed, the cleaning and drying of my chest cavity. Then in the midst of all the medical terminology was a short sentence he still chuckles about. "The chest cavity was cooled by dumping in a couple buckets of ice."

The description went on. My chest cavity was dried again. (I assume they removed the ice first or else I'll be "cold-hearted" for the rest of my life.) My new heart and lungs were put in place and sutured, and I was disconnected from the heart-lung machine. Dr. Reitz had put in the wires for a pacemaker, as is the rule in all heart transplants, as a precautionary measure. Fortunately they were never needed.

One line in the description of the operation puzzled Karl: the donor lungs had been "trimmed to fit." When Bruce came to see me, Karl asked him about it. Bruce told him the description was literally true. They had used scissors to trim the spongy lung tissues so they would fit precisely into my chest cavity. Karl shook his head and walked over to my bed and looked down at me.

I saw him and asked, "What do you want, Karl?"

"Nothing important now, Mary," he answered. "I'll tell you about it later."

There was nothing for Mother and Karl to do the first days after my surgery. The same cannot be said for the hospital personnel. A nurse was constantly in my room. If she had to take a break for any reason, another would relieve her. I needed constant monitoring and frequently needed medication. During the surgery they had put a shunt, an IV, into my jugular vein and another into my arm. Otherwise, within a few days, I would have been like a pincushion from all the needles. Every eight hours they took an X ray and an ECG. Several times a day a respiratory therapist would come in, sit me up, and pound on my back to try to get me to cough. I had fluid in my lungs and had to clear them to avoid danger of pneumonia. Also my lungs weren't fully expanded yet. That would take many weeks.

The respiration therapy made me extremely uncomfortable. As a result, I didn't try too hard. The therapists were at a loss, but Mother came up with a solution. She had them pull a tray table over to the bed so I could lean over it and get support while they pounded. Therapy went better after that.

I wasn't eating well. I needed calories to build tissue and make new blood. I knew it, everyone encouraged me, but I just couldn't get up an appetite. I picked at my food. Although Stanford is a wonderful hospital and I'll never tire of extolling its virtues, a gourmet's heaven it is not. Mother timidly asked Bruce Reitz if she could cook for me. Bruce agreed wholeheartedly. He hadn't wanted to ask her because he could see her knee was still very painful and she was having trouble getting around. But when Mother offered, he leaped on the idea.

The first meal she wanted to prepare was chicken soup with homemade noodles. I've always loved it, and Mother is a firm believer in the virtues of chicken soup. She sent Karl out with explicit instructions to find a chicken, not just any chicken, but a fat one. When he returned, the chicken wasn't fat enough, but she made it do.

I ate a little better after that but still not enough. The doctors wanted me to eat more. Was I getting enough calories to build the needed tissues? They were worried about my trachea where the lungs had been attached. Was it healing? They decided to take no chances and began feeding me intravenously in addition to my regular food. They started me on 5,000 calories a day.

My new lungs were working better, but they still hadn't fully expanded. In addition, they still retained some fluid, particularly on the right side. John Wallwork put a drain tube through my chest wall under my arm. I had been uncomfortable before. Now I couldn't even lie on my right side.

My joints, particularly my ankles, swelled from the steroids. They were inflamed and it was painful to stand or walk. I didn't mind that part. I didn't feel much like walking anyway. The doctors told us not to worry about the inflammation. It would go away when they were able to reduce the amount of steroids I was getting. Right now the larger danger was rejection. My body would react to the new organs as intruders and try to fight them off. The steroids and the cyclosporin A suppressed my immune system to prevent rejection. In time, the amounts I had to take could be reduced as my body built up a tolerance to the new organs, but for now I had to live with the side effects.

About ten days after my surgery, Mother arrived at the hospital to find me with a new complaint. Later, at breakfast, she said to my husband, "Karl, I think she is rejecting. I'm sure of it. Her feet are cold. Something is wrong."

On the way back to my room they met Bruce and John

Wallwork. Bruce and John were discussing the results of the biopsy Bruce had performed the day before. I had been taken back to the operating room where Bruce had gone in through my jugular vein and snipped off tiny pieces of my heart. The snippets were carefully analyzed under a microscope. Bruce told Karl the results of the analysis.

"We have found some early signs of rejection," Bruce said. "We don't think it's anything to worry about. We can handle it."

"Mother could have told you about the rejection," Karl said. "She told me about it at breakfast."

The doses of steroids were increased to fight the rejection. The list of medications was increased until even Karl lost track of what was what. Finally they decided to give me ATG, antithymocyte globulin, to combat the rejection. I had been warned about ATG before the surgery. It is the most painful shot imaginable. The nurses hate to give ATG. Even the Marquis de Sade would shrink from inflicting ATG on another human being. ATG isn't a single shot, but a series given in the thigh muscle. I had already had it, but that was right after my surgery when, blessedly, I was unconscious.

It was Tuesday, just over two weeks after my surgery, when Bruce ordered the ATG administered. The nurse brought in the three needles containing the ATG. They looked too big to give a horse let alone me. The nurse said to Mother, "I've got something she's not going to like."

I was still groggy from all the medication, but I think anyone who isn't afraid of the ATG would have to be dead. I asked Mother to hold my hand. The nurse administered the first shot. Suddenly Mother felt my hand go limp.

"Oh, my God!" Mother yelled. "Something's wrong!"

Instantly, the nurse put her stethoscope on my chest. The remaining needles scattered on the floor as she reached for the large red alarm button over my bed.

The result was instant action. Doctors and nurses appeared out of nowhere. John Wallwork was there so fast, Mother thought he must have been hiding under my bed. There was no panic, just action. Two people picked Mother up (she still couldn't move well) and carried her backward out of my room, across the hall, and into an office. Mother could see them working furiously over me, but she couldn't see what they were doing.

A nurse located Karl. He had been out in the waiting room having a cup of coffee. He came running down the hall. My room was so crowded that he couldn't have found a way in even if he had insisted. Karl joined Mother in the tiny office and did what he could to comfort her. There was little he could say; he was just as worried as she was. The two of them sat holding each other's hands. Mother kept repeating, "Oh, my God. She can't die. She's been through too much. She just can't die."

Mary Burge, a social worker for patients' families, and Lois Christopherson came to keep Mother and Karl company. I might not make it, and they wanted to be near to offer what help they could. In about twenty minutes, Bruce and John Wallwork appeared.

"We've got her breathing again" were Bruce's first words. "We have put her back on the ventilator for a while."

"She should be all right," John chimed in. "She didn't stop breathing long enough to do any permanent damage."

Karl knew what he meant. If my brain had been deprived of oxygen for too long I could have suffered brain damage. He didn't say anything. He nodded to John that he understood. Finally Karl asked the doctors, "What happened?"

"Too much fluid buildup," Bruce answered. "The rejection and some of the medications interfere with her kidneys. On top of that she has been getting a lot of fluids from the intravenous feeding. The fluids built up in her lungs, and it just became too hard for her to breathe.

"You see the lungs act like a pump for your kidneys. When your lungs don't work well, neither do your kidneys. In Mary's case, she couldn't breathe well because of the fluid in her lungs, which lowered her kidney function. The lowered kidney function caused more fluid to accumulate in her lungs. It became a vicious cycle until she stopped breathing."

They all came back to my room. Everyone was depressed. My condition had been stabilized, but now I seemed to be weaker than at any time since my surgery. I would have to start all over. For the rest of the day and on into the night not only my mother and Karl but also at least one of the doctors kept constant watch. They talked little. The only sound in the room was the soft hiss of the ventilator. I slept soundly.

The ventilator tube was taped to my mouth, and in addition, a catheter from my urinary tract emptied into a container alongside the bed. When my lungs began to work again, so did my kidneys. A slow but steady trickle of urine began to flow. My kidneys were pumping the excess fluid out of my body. At one point, John turned to Karl and said, "Did you ever think you would sit around and be glad to watch someone pee?" Karl laughed. John's humor broke the tension of the last hours. It needed breaking.

A few hours later, Karl called Max Jennings at the *Mesa Tribune* and told him about the incident. The news was picked up by the wire services and my story was again in newspapers all over the world. I felt a little embarrassed by all the attention, although I didn't realize its full extent at that time. All I had done was try to save my own life. I could see nothing heroic in that.

I remained on the ventilator for over twenty-four hours. The next day, before the tube was removed from my throat, Bruce used a bronchoscope to see how my trachea was healing. What he found was a relief to everyone—it was virtually healed. I had passed a giant hurdle on my road to recovery.

A week later Karl arrived at the hospital early, as he usually did, and sat by my bedside talking to me, trying to revive my interest in the world.

"Mary," he said, "today is twenty-four days since your transplant. Do you know you are now the longest-living heart-lung transplant?"

I nodded. I really didn't care about setting records. I had suffered a setback, I was still rejecting, I was still having trouble eating, I still felt like hell, but I was alive. I knew that much. They could keep their records. I was just happy to be alive.

THIRTEEN

AFTER I CAME OFF THE VENTILATOR THE SECOND TIME AND started to breathe on my own, the doctors remained concerned. I was still rejecting the new organs. They continued to administer heavy doses of steroids, as well as other drugs. The side effects of the drugs built up and began to affect my mind. I became somewhat paranoid. My room was separated from the corridor by glass walls, and as people walked by, they would look into my room. I felt like a goldfish in a bowl. People were watching me.

As part of my morning routine, the nurse would draw samples of blood from the tube in my neck for analysis. One morning, as the nurse started to take the blood, I snapped at her, "You're not going to do it! Get out! I'm going home."

The startled nurse smiled at me. "Mary, you're not going home today."

"Yes I am!" I told her firmly. "The helicopter from Williams Field is here. You're not taking any blood."

My nurse summoned her relief. Maybe she would have better luck with me.

"Mary, I have to take your blood," she said calmly.

Her luck with me was no better. "Forget it!" I snapped at her. I hadn't forgotten how to fight. "I'm going home today. Get my clothes. They're waiting for me. In fact, get me the phone."

The telephone was sitting on top of the defibrillator, which was in the room at all times. The nurse handed the phone to me, I suppose to calm me. By this time, I was having trouble with my memory. I had complained to Karl that I couldn't even remember how to spell three-letter words. But when the nurse handed me the phone, I sat up and dialed the number of our Palo Alto apartment on the first try.

Mother answered groggily. It was 5:30 A.M.

"Mother."

"Mary, what's wrong?"

Mother was astonished. I sounded perfectly lucid, but what did I want at that hour of the morning?

"Put Karl on the phone," I ordered.

When Karl answered, I said, "Where the hell are you? You'd better get over here because the helicopter is here to take me home and you're not here."

"You're going home today?" Karl asked. He tried not to sound surprised.

"Yes, so get over here. I told the nurse to have your coffee ready."

"Okay," Karl said, matter-of-factly. "I'll be there in a minute."

I hung up the phone and told the nurse, "I told Karl you would have his coffee ready." I still refused to let anyone take blood.

Neither Karl nor anyone else could drink coffee in my room. It was impossible to drink coffee through the masks they all wore. The nurse didn't point out that obvious fact to me. She got a cup of coffee.

When Karl arrived ten minutes later he sat down to talk to me. I had forgotten all about the imaginary helicopter. "You're here early today," I said.

Karl nodded and smiled at me. The nurse took the blood samples.

In the days that followed I continued to hallucinate.

Once I called Karl, early in the morning, and asked him to rush to the hospital. When he arrived, I had him sit close to me so I could talk to him without the nurse hearing.

"Karl," I whispered, "you've got to get me out of here. They are murdering the patients. I saw them last night. They buried one right out in the hall."

Karl held my hand and assured me that he wouldn't let anything happen to me.

Both Mother and Karl were worried about my continuing hallucinations. Karl asked John Wallwork about them.

"I know what's wrong with her," John answered. "She's bloody crazy."

He went on to explain that my condition wasn't at all unusual. The combination of major surgery, steroids, and the confinement often caused paranoia in patients. They were glad it wasn't worse. Sometimes patients got the idea they were being poisoned and wouldn't eat or take the needed medications. The hallucinations would pass when they could reduce my medications.

In the days that followed, however, I began to have a recurring dream. At first I told no one about it, but finally I could keep my fears to myself no longer. I told Karl. Again and again I dreamed of one of the consent forms I had signed before the operation. Somehow it became distorted in my mind.

"Karl," I told him. "The transplant didn't work. They are going to do it again. They won't let me die. They are going to do it again and again. They are going to keep me here, operating and operating. I want you to find out how to get hold of the Mafia. Hire them to come and murder me."

Another time I told him to get a lawyer and force them to let me die. Hallucinating or not, I was serious, and Karl listened quietly and tried to reassure me. He humored me, but he was worried. He told Bruce about my dreams.

The problem was resolved one day when I suddenly asked Bruce, "What would happen if I died?"

"Then you would be dead," Bruce said evenly. "We would bury you."

"You wouldn't do anything else to me?"

"There wouldn't be anything else we could do," Bruce answered gently. "You would be dead."

"You wouldn't bring me back to life and do this all over again?" I asked.

"No," Bruce said, smiling at me. "One to a customer."

His answer reassured me. My dreams stopped after that. The rejection finally began to resolve, and they were able to reduce the steroids. As John had predicted, my sanity returned.

I continued to receive mail from all over the world. For some reason my plight had caught the public imagination. Mail came from a cross section of people and was uniformly uplifting. I received mail from housewives, people in the media, people in business, retired people. I received cards from grade-school classes. Later, on Mother's Day, cards came from a third-grade class at a California school. One of the children had heard I was a mother. Much of the mail came from people who were ill and who somehow managed to find inspiration in my story.

One of the first letters was from Jack Mathes, a captain for United Airlines.

"Your gutsiness is a zinging inspiration to all of us!" he wrote. "We'll be thinking fondly, and proudly, of you from 39,000 feet. Infinite cheer!"

Captain Mathes would be one of the few letter writers I would meet, although at the time he wrote, it seemed like a long shot indeed.

A radio newsman, George Bryant, from station KNCR in Fortuna, California, wrote: "Just before your surgery, we reported news of you and your illness. Our listeners flooded our phone lines and asked that we send their feelings on to you. Humboldt County people are moved greatly by your courage."

The idea of my courage was a redundant theme in many of the letters. Some of the letters were touching.

They left me with a feeling of awe and a little guilt. I couldn't see where I had done anything so courageous and inspiring.

An anonymous writer told me, "I am impressed and rejuvenated by your courage. I work daily with people who are constantly trying to destroy themselves (drug addicts) and have been feeling very burned out after four years. But your extraordinary optimism and spirit have really given my recent cynicism about humanity a good kick in the pants. I was glad to read of someone who loves life enough to fight for it. . . . I am equally in awe of the love and bravery shown not only by your family, but by Ofelia Jones. . . . " It was one of the few letters to mention the donor's mother.

Mother liked the letters from schoolchildren most. Reading them was one of the few things that cheered her days and made them go faster. Sometimes they came in packets, class assignments. Once in a while the writer made it painfully obvious that he or she was writing under orders. Included in a packet from St. Clements School in Hayward, California, one note read, "We had to write you a letter, but I hope you are feeling better." Michelle McDonald wrote, "We have been praying for you every day. And I think God will touch you and you will live until you are 81 years old. . . . I have a lizard named Toot, and when I told him you were O.K. he sang the most beautiful song you ever heard. I guess he was happy for you too."

One of Michelle's classmates decided to fill me in on the news at his home: "I am 10 and in the fourth grade. I have a dog and three cats."

I received a card or letter from my family back in Buffalo at least once, sometimes twice, a day. My brother Bill Erickson had married since I had left Buffalo and I had never met his wife, Denise. Denise wrote, "Love you, love you, love you, love you, love you, love you, love you, love you, XOXOXOXOXOXOXOXOXOXOXOXOXO. That should be enough for one day."

Mother would show me each card and read every letter to me. She tried to arouse my interest, but she could not. I was withdrawn and too filled with my own troubles and fears to pay any attention. It would be months before I found enough strength to appreciate the caring and sentiments people were showing for me. At best, I was a bit embarrassed by all the attention.

Karl and Mother were worried by my attitude. I didn't even want to get out of bed. Part of the time I was psychologically unbalanced by all the medication, or as John Wallwork bluntly put it, "bloody crazy." Drugs weren't the only cause, however. I was becoming used to being a patient. It was easier to have things done than to do them. I became an expert at manipulation. I always figured out an excuse for what I wanted and I was very obstinate. I had physical therapy every day, so I would think of some way to avoid it.

"My leg hurts. I don't feel up to it. I'm too tired." I'd tell them anything.

The nurses knew what I was doing up to a point, but they had no experience to guide them. They had no way of knowing how strong I really was, so they were reluctant to push me too hard. I was sneaky; I knew their dilemma and used it. Strangely enough, I knew what I was doing and hated myself for doing it, but I just couldn't stop. I had always assumed that after my operation I would be a star. I'd get up and walk out of the hospital faster than anyone else had dreamed. That had been my self-image and what I had promised myself before the operation. I was disgusted with myself, and I guess my disgust explains why I didn't want to hear all the letters Mother read to me. I felt I was failing myself, and the expressions of admiration from those kind people made me feel I was failing them too. I didn't want to be reminded of it.

Mother and Karl weren't the only ones who worried about my attitude; my nurses and doctors did too. I had to start getting up and doing things for myself. I needed to recover my strength. Bruce knew me better than I thought. He brought out his trump card. He had a nurse, Chris Craig, reassigned to my case.

Bruce knew Chris and I would get along. But he knew something else: Chris wouldn't let me get away with being a petty tyrant. For the rest of my life I'll be thankful to Chris for what she did for me. Chris was a fiery, redheaded Scot, prone to swearing, gentle, yet tough as nails. Chris would take grief from no one, least of all her newly famous patient. She wasn't much bigger than I, a five-foot-three stringbean, very pretty, but never wearing a trace of makeup. We locked wills almost immediately. I tried, at the beginning, to gain a few concessions from Chris, but I got nowhere.

Chris worked days, and her standard greeting when she came on shift was to sweep into my room, throw her arms around me, and proclaim, "Are you all right my wee bonny baby?"

I was always glad to see her and would often answer, "Yes."

"Then get your bloody ass out of bed."

I'd get.

One day Chris came in with a new project. "Mary," she began, "I'll tell you what we're going to do tomorrow. We're going to wash your hair. It's a mess. You'll feel better when it's clean. I'll bring in my blow-dryer and shampoo."

I was not impressed by her idea. "I don't want my hair washed," I told her.

"Well, you're going to get your hair washed," Chris promised. "Don't worry about it."

True to her word, Chris showed up the next day with a large brown bag. Out of the bag she brought shampoo, creme rinse, her hair dryer, and a big black plastic garbage bag.

"Come on, now, my wee baby, get out of that bed," Chris ordered.

I stood up while Chris disconnected the ECG wires, my oxygen, and the various other paraphernalia I wore. She punched a hole in the bag for my head, none for my arms, and pulled it over my head, then helped me over to the sink.

"Come on. Bend over at the waist," Chris demanded. "We're going to get your hair washed."

"My chest hurts," I complained.

"We're not going to wash your bloody chest."

I felt violated, standing there with my arms pinned to my sides by the bag, my head poking out the hole at the top. "This isn't the way to do it," I argued.

"Well, this is the way it's going to be done," Chris said firmly. "You've got to get your hair washed." She bent me over the sink and began to try to adjust the water temperature with the foot pedals below. It was awkward to say the least. Water splashed everywhere.

"I'm getting wet," I protested.

"Don't worry about it; I've got towels on the floor."

I wasn't worried about the damned floor. "But I'm freezing," I protested again.

Chris ignored my protests, shampooed vigorously, and finally rinsed it out. I was relieved; my ordeal was over. Then, to my horror, she slapped on more shampoo.

"What are you doing?" I demanded.

"A lady always shampoos twice. That's the way I was taught and you're going to be a lady."

I wasn't interested in being a lady. "My chest hurts," I complained again.

"Shut up!"

There was little else I could do, so I was quiet. Chris finished shampooing me, put on the creme rinse, and rinsed that off. Finally she released me from my garbage bag prison, dried me off, and smiled as she wrapped me in a prewarmed blanket.

Then Chris got out her blow-dryer and proceeded to dry my hair, singing one of her happy Scottish ballads as she did so.

"Who gives a shit about your damned Scottish song?" I

asked glumly. I did like it, but I was feeling bitter at the way I was being treated.

My bitterness didn't bother Chris in the least. "Just be quiet," she answered. "You're going to look beautiful."

It was the kind of scene that took place many times between us. I still had to be x-rayed every day, but the staff no longer brought the portable unit to my room. Chris insisted I walk at least part of the way to X ray. She would let me take the wheelchair, but I had to push it.

I did win one small battle with Chris. I suffer from mild claustrophobia, and anytime I left my isolation room I had to dress in the gown, booties, gloves, the whole works. I didn't like it, but except for the mask, I could stand it. The mask was genuinely too much for me. I'd start to panic whenever I wore it and couldn't wait to get back to my room. I insisted that if I had to wear it I wouldn't leave my room. Chris talked to Bruce Reitz, and he decided it was more important that I exercise than wear the mask. I could go out without it, and everyone would cross their fingers that I wouldn't pick up an infection.

Karl took a few days to go home and see the boys. My son Chris had left Palo Alto about a week after my surgery and was home alone, taking care of both himself and the house. Luke was still staying at the home of my former boss, Haney Womack. Karl talked to the boys nearly every day on the phone, but he wanted to see them, to be sure they were all right, and to reassure them I was OK.

He found Chris to be a remarkably good housekeeper. Everything at home was in shape. Lucas was his usual ebullient self. Karl went into work for a few days to check the progress of a project he had started, a design of some equipment for a Canadian telephone company. His boss had taken over his work, but Karl felt compelled to give everything the once-over. Fortunately, Comtech Data Corporation continued to send his paychecks the entire time he was with me at Stanford. They were all the income we had at the time. I had quit the newspaper the previous

September and my disability payments didn't begin for six months.

After a few days at home, Karl had satisfied himself that everything was okay there. He decided to come back to Stanford. I needed him more than he was needed in Mesa. The people at Comtech told him to take off and not to worry about work. The doors would still be open when I recovered. He came back to Palo Alto.

FOURTEEN

I HAD A BLISTER ON THE BALL OF MY FOOT. WHEN KARL returned from Arizona, he found this to be my most serious problem. I had finally started to walk up and down the hall outside my room. I was always assisted by at least one nurse who carefully watched over me and pushed the IV bottles along as I walked. Walking was no fun. It was hard, and I still didn't want to see anybody, or more accurately, I didn't want to be seen. The blister made things worse. Now it was genuinely painful to take a step.

Dr. Reitz viewed my blister as a major problem because he wanted me to keep walking. He was not going to take any kind of chance with any kind of infection. Because of my severely suppressed immune system, an infected blister was a potential catastrophe. I only knew that my foot hurt when I walked on it. Bruce called in a dermatologist.

Mother shared my sentiments about my blister. I was impatient with all the consultations, which seemed to accomplish nothing. I called the group of doctors my "blister committee."

I asked the blister committee, "You can take out a heart and lungs and do all this fancy work, but why does it take four doctors and a Philadelphia lawyer to figure out what to do about a damned blister?"

"Well," Bruce defended, "we have to be very careful that infection doesn't set in."

After the second or third conference on my blister over a period of several days, Bruce and the dermatologist huddled in the corner so I couldn't hear them while they talked. They came over to announce what they would be doing: nothing. Mother listened incredulously, but said not a word. After the doctors left, she went down to the hospital drugstore and bought a bottle of Campho-Phenique and some cotton swabs.

Mother respected the doctors' opinions and their expertise when it came to things like transplant surgery, which were almost beyond her comprehension, but she had seen blisters, fever blisters, cuts, and the like all her life. They weren't something you went to a doctor about; she knew how to take care of them and she knew what worked. She applied the Campho-Phenique to my blister every few hours. In a couple of days, as Mother knew it would, my blister dried up and went away.

I began to make slow but steady progress during my second month after surgery. Each day I grew almost imperceptibly stronger and I could walk a little better. I still had to be encouraged to walk and I still wanted to avoid meeting people. But Chris Craig wouldn't take no for an answer, and since the other nurses now knew I could do it, neither would they. Mother and Karl encouraged me. Karl in particular was puzzled by my reluctance to do anything but lie in bed. He knew from our talks before the surgery that I had been determined to get back on my feet as soon as possible. My actions seemed out of character to him, but he said little about his concerns. He was relieved that I was finally making progress. Then I had my second serious setback.

My doctors still aren't sure what happened. It may

have been the aspirin they had been giving me for the pain I was experiencing in my knees. Whatever it was, one of the medications apparently triggered rectal bleeding. It became worse and worse until it was a serious problem. Blood transfusions were prescribed to counteract the blood loss. I still grew weaker and had to stop walking outside my room. I stopped taking the aspirin, but it would be more than three weeks before the bleeding would end and I could again make any progress in gaining my strength.

The setback caused by the bleeding was not revealed to the public. Both the hospital staff and I wanted to avoid any more attention from the media than we could help. Every morning since my surgery the hospital public relations staff had informed Karl what statements would be made that day about my case. My family tried to hold contacts with the media to a minimum. Revealing the story of my bleeding problems seemed to smack of sensationalism to me, and that I didn't want.

Nevertheless, the story continued hot. In some ways my notoriety was difficult for me. People walking down the hall outside my glass-walled room almost always looked in. They would smile and often give a friendly wave to me. Every time I walked the halls of the hospital, people would come up and wish me well or talk to me. It wasn't that I didn't appreciate their concern and good wishes, but I missed my privacy and anonymity. The fact that I was very withdrawn only made the problem worse.

I still slept much of the time. Frequently I had to be awakened during the day to take medicine or to eat. I continued to show little interest in my surroundings. I had always been an avid reader, but now I didn't even want to read. Karl had bought me two books I had asked for before my surgery, and they still lay, unread, on the table alongside my bed. I had trouble keeping my mind on anything. When I tried to read, my attention would wander after a few words.

Although my hallucinations had gone away when the doctors were able to reduce my medications, I was still having psychological problems. Before my surgery, as my lungs began to fail, I had begun to take oxygen. I could feel some strength returning when I did so. After my surgery, I continued to take oxygen much of the time. At first, I needed it, but as my lungs grew stronger, my need ended. I still wanted the oxygen. Intellectually I knew why my doctors wanted me to give it up, but I couldn't. They began to reduce slowly the amount of oxygen I was getting. I didn't like that idea at all. I complained to Bruce, who finally decided to restore it. "One of these days she'll get sick of it and give it up," he said. "It's not hurting anything."

My reaction was, in many ways, typical of people who spend long periods in intensive care. Typical or not, it was hard on my family. At times, Karl could not understand me. I was often irritable and would blow up at the slightest thing. For example, when I had started to bleed again, I was allowed to ride in a wheelchair down for my morning X ray. As I improved, it was a constant battle to get me to walk again. One day, Karl came in and asked me, "Did you walk to X ray today?"

I blew up. "Can't you ever say anything else? What are you doing? Checking up on me?" I hurt Karl's feelings. He couldn't understand what was wrong.

My condition preyed on my mind. Early one morning when Karl arrived, I asked him in a soft voice, "Karl, could you come over here by the bed for a minute?"

"Sure, hon," he replied, pulling a chair over beside my bed.

"I have been thinking all night," I began. "I have come to the conclusion that as long as we are married, I will never get well. I will die in the hospital. That's why we have to get a divorce."

Karl was stunned. I hadn't been hallucinating and sounded entirely lucid. He said if that was what I needed, he would take care of it. In a short time, he left my room and went to see my doctors and Lois Christopherson. They all shrugged it off.

"At the moment," Bruce told him, "she may mean it. But it'll pass. It may be hours, it may be a few days."

Karl was not particularly comforted.

"Why don't you take off for a couple of days?" Lois suggested.

Karl went back to the apartment and was packing a suitcase when Mother found him.

"What are you doing?" she asked. "Where are you going?"

Karl told her what happened.

"Well, why don't you just go up and see your mother for a few days?" she suggested. Karl's mother lived only a few hours away and he decided that's what he would do. He drove my mother back to the hospital to drop her off before leaving town. He was depressed. It was the second time I had rejected him. In a macabre way, the reason was the same in both instances. I felt I was doing what I had to do to take care of myself.

When Mother and Karl pulled up in front of the hospital, I was there waiting for them. I'd had Chris bring me down in a wheelchair. Mother got out of the car, walked over, and kissed me on the cheek. I had already forgotten what I had said to Karl earlier and was surprised when he started to back the car away.

Mother didn't know what to say. Finally she told me, "Karl's going up to visit his mother for a couple of days."

"Well, tell him not to go anywhere," I insisted. "I want him to stay here."

Mother flagged Karl down and walked over to the car. "Karl, go park the car and get back here. She doesn't remember anything."

When Karl returned, I scolded him. "Why would you go off to visit your mother without telling me?"

Karl smiled at me. He felt better.

Karl wasn't the only victim of my ill temper. No one was immune. A couple of days later my mother was subjected to the same kind of fire. She came into my room to find me in bed, staring at the ceiling.

"What are you going to do? Lie there all day?" Mother chided. "Why don't you get dressed?"

I became furious. "Mother, don't you tell me what to do! I know how I feel. When I want to get my clothes on and go, I will. But I don't feel like it. I'm not up to it. I'm tired."

Mother retreated, her feelings bruised.

I didn't understand myself either. I knew I was acting irrationally, at least part of the time, and it troubled me. I didn't know if the cause was the medication, the operation, the long convalescence, or what, but I was learning a new dimension of myself and I didn't like it. I spent a lot of time thinking such things as, "Okay, I'm alive. I made it. Now, what's the next step?" The question bothered me. I didn't have an answer. I have always been a believer in controlling my own destiny, and suddenly the miracle of my survival had little meaning because I had nothing to look forward to. All I ever seemed to feel was tired. In one of my more rational moments I told Karl of my feelings and wondered where my strength had gone.

"You used it up," he said. "You had to fight so hard to stay alive through the operation that you used what strength you had. Now you have to find more. Don't worry, you will."

I appreciated his confidence, even if I didn't share it. No one knew where I was going to find this added strength. I continued to worry.

Audrey Covner, my primary-care nurse, and I had become close personal friends during my long stay in intensive care. Audrey, a pretty woman in her mid-twenties, was cheerful and gentle, in many ways the opposite of the fiery Scot, Chris Craig. I idolized both of them.

One night, I had a particularly bad episode of rectal

bleeding. Audrey cleaned up both me and the bed. It was 2 A.M., and the two of us were alone in the quiet room.

When she finished cleaning up, Audrey asked me, "Can I do anything else for you?"

"Would you sit and hold my hand?" I asked. "I'm afraid." Audrey Covner was the first person I ever uttered those words to.

Audrey took my hand in hers. "What are you afraid of?" she asked softly. "Do you want to talk about it?"

"I don't know. It seems I'm afraid of everything. Where am I going from here? What am I going to do?" I wept. Audrey was still sitting, holding my hand, when I went to sleep.

In spite of all my problems, I continued to make progress. For the first time since my surgery, I began to grow curious about the world outside the narrow confines of my intensive-care room. I wondered what was happening in my old advertising department at the *Mesa Tribune.* One day, on impulse, I called my oldest friend at the paper, Joyce Howland. Joyce was astonished by my unexpected call. Word spread quickly, and before the call was over, I had talked to more than a dozen people. I hung up the phone, exhausted but happy for a change. I was thinking about something other than myself.

The doctors began gradually to reduce the restrictions of my isolation. It was a joyous moment when I could see people again without their having to wear those depressing green gowns and caps, when I could feel the touch of a human hand without rubber gloves. The nurses were instructed to leave me alone, only for a few minutes at first but gradually for longer periods.

I began to visit the transplant clinic where I would see my doctors after I was released from the hospital. I hoped to be able to go home in a few months, but I would have to return to Stanford in January for my first set of tests. If they showed that everything was okay I would not have to come back for a year unless my doctor at home thought I needed to go back. The transplant program was doing so well that most of us only had to come back once a year. Most problems that might arise, such as infections, could be taken care of by our local doctors. The prospect of checkups only once a year was encouraging because the emphasis was on quality living and not illness.

I was encouraged to get to know other transplant patients. Some still lived in the Stanford area, and some came back to Stanford for their yearly checkups. One man, an advertising executive, was now working in a music store. Another was writing a cookbook. It occurred to me that the people I met were living new lives, doing things they had never done before. I was frightened by the prospect. I thought, "Where am I going to go from here? What am I going to do?" I kept my thoughts to myself. It would be a long time before I could share my feelings with anyone.

There were several heart transplant patients in my wing, all of them men. The thing I noticed the most in conversations with them was that they were all extremely worried about how they would cope with the future and earn a living. Many were concerned about whether they could continue to be the head of the family. I don't think any of them really levelled with me about this. They kept up a front, but they were fearful to a man about losing their self respect.

It made me think, "My God, am I going to be able to go back to my job and do my work like I used to? Will there be a place for me?" All of us seemed to be looking for our place. We were different, no matter how much we wanted to think otherwise. In this respect, I was like all of them.

The man who was writing the cookbook—I can't remember his name any longer—had a wonderful sense of humor. His little girl, who he loved dearly, came to see him often, always clutching a teddy bear to whom she pretended to administer cyclosporin. She couldn't have been more than six, but she could rattle off the names of the drugs her daddy was taking.

When her father would talk to me in quiet moments after the family left, he told me he was writing the cookbook so he could make money. Being able to earn money was the most important thing to him at that time. I think it was more difficult in that respect for the male transplant patients than it was for me. Sure, I wanted to be productive again, but my identity wasn't completely wrapped up in that.

One day, Bruce walked into my room and announced matter-of-factly, "Mary, we're going to move you to the third floor."

I panicked. He might as well have said he was going to torture me. I knew that when transplant patients moved to the third floor they had to start doing things for themselves. I was already taking care of all my medications; no transplant patient can leave intensive care until he or she can manage that much. I was sure I could not survive on the third floor. They might take away my oxygen.

Bruce ignored my objections, and I was moved the next day. Chris Craig, whom I often called my "drill sergeant," became very emotional the day I left NICU. She blustered around my room, packing my things, and finally burst into tears. I wasn't surprised. I knew Chris genuinely liked me, and I felt the same way about her. Ours was more than a nurse-patient relationship. Life on the third floor without Chris would be missing a lot. Through her tears, Chris reassured me. "You'll be all right. I'll be up to see you every day." She admonished the nurses on the third floor, "Now you take good care of her."

Fifteen minutes later Chris was back in my new room.

"It's not night yet," I said to her. "You said you would be back tonight."

"Are you sure you're all right?" Chris asked. "Do you have everything you need?"

I looked around the new room. I decided I didn't like it. I should have. There were no glass walls, and I had a door and could enjoy some privacy for a change, which I had been craving for weeks. The heart-monitoring equipment, the familiar defibrillator, and the ventilator that had been alongside my bed were gone. There was no shelf of drugs to be used in emergencies. The absence of equipment was a tangible sign that the doctors no longer believed my life was in immediate danger. I was becoming more and more an ordinary patient recovering from surgery. The changes should have made me glad, but they didn't. I was afraid.

Chris came back to see me on her break and again before she left for the evening. Several other nurses from the second-floor NICU dropped in to say good night. Audrey visited the next morning. For the rest of my stay on the third floor some of the nurses from NICU would drop in to see me regularly.

I sensed that some of the third-floor nurses resented me and the special consideration I received from my friends from intensive care. I think they assumed from all the press coverage that I was some sort of a prima donna. I didn't consider myself special and was hurt by their attitude. Still, I understood that it was important for me to become more independent.

The day I moved to the third floor, Bruce Reitz and Audrey Covner, my primary-care nurse, prepared the third-floor staff with a special briefing on my case, emphasizing the differences between my case and that of a normal heart transplant patient. Audrey had written a manual on the care of heart-lung transplant patients. I suppose the special briefing didn't help my cause.

I was still having a problem with rectal bleeding. There was little the doctors could do except take me off the aspirin and give me transfusions. I had to take prednisone, which carries the side effect of making you into a bleeder. I couldn't give it up or I would reject my new organs. I was lucky in some ways because the cyclosporin A drastically reduces the amount of prednisone you need.

After I had been on the third floor about ten days, I

was allowed to go home to our apartment for a few hours. Bruce drove me to the apartment; perhaps he wanted to be there to deal with any last-minute reservations on my part. Mother had fixed one of my favorite meals, liver and onions, and she bustled around the apartment while I rested. The short ride to the apartment had exhausted me. A few hours later, a nurse came over to rinse the shunt in my neck with heparin to keep it from clotting. Her visit served to remind me just how dependent on medical and nursing attention I still was.

When I returned to the hospital that evening, the only thing I wanted to do was get my clothes off and get into bed. My nurses weren't surprised, but I was astonished at the extent of my exhaustion. It was a realistic reminder of how far I still had to go.

About a week later, Bruce walked into my room and told me, "We're going to release you in two days."

I didn't know whether to be happy or frightened. I opted for frightened. I knew as well as my doctors did that I was becoming so emotionally dependent on the hospital environment that it was restricting my progress. I was unwilling to do things for myself, things I needed to do. Mother was frightened by Bruce's announcement too. She was afraid of having to care for me by herself. Bruce Reitz gave us no option. He wanted me out of the hospital.

The day for my release arrived. Our first stop on the way out was the hospital cafeteria. Mother had given the chef her solemn promise we would stop in before we left. Bruce, Mother, and I waited at the table while John Wallwork bought coffee and collected forks. He returned and sat at attention, fork pointing upward, waiting like a small boy for the expected cake.

The chef appeared at our table with a box, which he opened for our inspection. It contained a lovely hand-embroidered tablecloth. I loved it immediately, and it still looks beautiful on my dining room table. I was thrilled and thanked the chef both for the gift and for the meals he had prepared during the previous three months. Unfortunately, John wasn't equally thrilled. He had expected a cake, and John loves cake. One glance at his ample girth will attest to that. The disappointment was written on his face.

Bruce laughed.

"What are you upset about? Good surgeons shouldn't be fat," he chided John. Bruce, tall, lean and strong, frequently kidded John about his weight.

We started toward the front entrance of the hospital. Mother, having gone ahead of the rest of us, came hurrying back.

"My God," she said. "Look at the crowd out there!"

I could see nothing, I was too far from the door as yet, but Bruce and John took a look. When they came back, Bruce said, "She can't go out that way." The front of the hospital was mobbed with reporters, photographers, TV newsmen, and other media people.

"We'll take her out the back," Bruce continued, turning my wheelchair around.

I was disappointed—not at avoiding the media; I really didn't feel up to facing them that day. But I had entered the hospital through the front door, almost three months earlier, and it seemed important to me that I leave the same way. Still, Bruce was right; I didn't have the strength to run that gauntlet. Besides, there would be a news conference in two days; the media would get their story then.

We left through the back exit, past the loading dock. "This is great," I said. "Ducking out between the garbage cans."

A hospital security guard had brought a car to take us to the apartment, and Bruce's little red car had been brought around too. Bruce and John took a few pictures, then Mother and I piled into the car for the mile ride home. Bruce followed in his car to see that I was all right.

When we arrived at the apartment, the guard helped me out and up the elevator to our fourth-floor apartment.

As Mother unlocked the door, I remembered the evening, nearly three months earlier, when we had left. At that time, I had wondered what was ahead. Now that was behind me. I had lived and was free of the hospital at last. I little dreamed what a long road lay ahead.

FIFTEEN

EARLY JUNE IN PALO ALTO WAS BEAUTIFUL. MAYBE IT ALWAYS is, but it seemed especially wonderful to me—almost as if the world were saying, "Welcome back, Mary." I loved it. The temperature in Mesa usually reaches the hundred-degree mark in late May and stays there. I hate going outside in summer at home; it's too hot. In the soft, warm, late spring of northern California, going out was a pleasure.

Mother and I went out frequently, window-shopping mostly; our family finances didn't allow much else. Sometimes we would stop for lunch. Everywhere we went, I was recognized. Most of the time people would walk up to me and say something like, "How are you doing, Mary?" They would invariably follow, sometimes without waiting for my answer, with "You're great" or "I can't tell you how wonderful you are."

I couldn't understand their attitude. I hadn't done anything great. All I had done was find, partly by accident, a chance to save my life and to take that chance. Their accolades should have been given to Bruce Reitz. He performed the transplant operation. He put years of his life into finding a way to save the lives of others. Those were great and wonderful achievements. I had simply become ill with a terminal disease, and I surely didn't try to bring that about. I often said to Mother, after my well-wishers had left, "Why do these people make such a fuss over my operation? Thousands of people have operations every day. Why should I be treated any differently?"

One day at lunch, I noticed three women sitting at a nearby table staring at me. One of them finally got up and came over to our table.

"I don't want to intrude on your lunch," she said, "but are you Mary?"

"Yes, I am."

"I'm happy to see you out of the hospital. You look good."

I would have one version or another of that conversation hundreds of times over the next few months. Universally, the people who came up to me were kind and sincere. Most addressed me by my first name, as if we were old friends. I never minded their familiarity. Somehow it made their kindness more personal. I have never forgotten the attitude of people toward me. I had not known there was so much compassion in the world.

When I left the hospital, I knew I would have to stay in the Palo Alto area for several months. I, like all transplant recipients, visited the Stanford clinic three times a week for blood tests and X rays. I still often saw Bruce Reitz, but as a clinic patient, I had a new cardiologist, Dr. Sharon Hunt. Sharon performed my biopsies to check on rejection and handled my day-to-day medical problems. All signs of rejection had long since disappeared, and Sharon reduced the amount of prednisone and cyclosporin A I had to take. I didn't mind. My new heart and lungs were fine.

One day as we were leaving the hospital, five middle-aged women in a beatup car were pulling out of the parking lot. When they spotted me, they acted as if they had seen a movie star. They began to honk the horn, and two of them stuck their hands out the window, waving wildly, "Hey Mary! Hang in there! You're doing great!" The car roared off, leaving Mother and me standing there, smiling.

While I had been in the hospital, I had been protected from the media, but now I was out and would finally have to meet them. Max Jennings, the executive editor of the *Mesa Tribune* and the man whose efforts had helped me stay alive, had warned me what to expect.

"Mary, you'll be asked some tough questions. It's their job to get information, not to be nice to you."

As it turned out, Max wasn't completely correct. I had my first news conference a few days after I left the hospital, and I found the media very nice. I'm not sure how much information they got, but they weren't tough.

On the day of that first news conference, the hospital had arranged for Chuck Walker and me to talk to a few pool reporters from the networks and the wire services. Chuck was the second heart-lung transplant and hadn't yet been released from the hospital.

On the day of the press conference, I woke up with a sinus infection and was feeling lousy. I even suggested delaying it. Mother would have no part of that idea. "All the reporters will be there!" she scolded. I reluctantly decided to go through with it.

When we arrived at the hospital, Mrs. Kennedy, the wife of the president of Stanford University, greeted me with a kiss on the cheek and gave me a wicker basket filled with lovely flowers. It was a long walk to the interview room, and because I was feeling so rotten, I took a wheelchair ride to face the newsmen. Chuck Walker was there before me, and together we didn't get a single surprising or embarrassing question. They asked how we felt, what we would do when we got home, all the simple, predictable things.

Max could never understand why they treated me so gently, why they seemed to back off from tackling the really tough issues. I was comfortable with the press. They were my people too. I knew my way around a newsroom. Maybe that explained part of their gentle treatment. Maybe part of it was that I tried to give answers that were straightforward and direct. The reporters didn't feel I was trying to dodge anything, and I wasn't. I think they understood something of what we had been through; they respected our ordeal and didn't want to add to our problems.

The pleasant days of June passed easily. I was slowly gaining strength and becoming acclimatized to life outside the hospital. I finally reached one milestone. I got rid of my oxygen. I had feared moving to the third floor at the hospital because I might have to give up the oxygen, but I had it there. Before I was discharged, Karl arranged for oxygen at the apartment so I would have it there. Every night, before I went to bed, I carefully set the flow and put the tube into my nose. One night, I awoke with the tube around my neck, my nose and throat dry from the oxygen. I said to myself, "This is stupid!" I shut the oxygen off. Bruce had been right when he said not to worry. The time had come when I was ready to give it up and I did.

Then, without warning, tragedy struck. My aunt Lorraine, Mother's younger sister, died. She and Mother had lived together in Florida for years. When I was a child, I had idolized Lorraine. I had thought her the most beautiful girl alive, and she loved to spoil me. I had talked to her regularly since I had been out of the hospital, the last time only a few days before her death. Now she was gone and I was too weak even to go to her funeral.

Mother was worried. In addition to her grief, she didn't want to leave me alone. I assured her there was no danger in leaving me; besides, Karl could come up if necessary.

I hated to see Karl take off more time from work. Comtech had been so good to us already that I hated to take advantage of their generosity. Fortunately, Karl didn't have to return to Palo Alto. Two old friends, John Hanron and his wife Cheryl, had moved to the Bay area. John had been my assistant at the paper and had recently moved to California. Cheryl had also worked at the *Mesa Tribune* and when, the previous fall, they had told Karl and me they were getting married we were happy for both of them. Their wedding was one of the many things I missed due to my illness. John and Cheryl offered to look in on me so I wouldn't be alone. From then on, while I was in Palo Alto, I could be sure of seeing at least one of them every week and Cheryl called almost daily to see how I was and if I needed anything. Mostly I was just glad to hear a familiar voice or see the face of an old friend.

Karl, Chris, and Luke came up over the Fourth of July weekend. It was the first time I had seen them since leaving the hospital. They were disappointed when they arrived. I was back in the hospital. I had developed a blister on my back, although this time the doctors didn't wonder what it was; it was herpes. They weren't surprised. Transplant recipients often develop herpes infections as a result of their depressed immune systems. In fact, many of the infections we develop are caused by viruses we, like everyone, carry with us. They are kept under control by the body's normal defense mechanisms. After a transplant, those defenses are suppressed and the infection shows up.

I was in the hospital a week before they got the herpes under control. By then, Mother had returned.

Mother had a new idea. We should take a vacation for a few days. Mother loves to gamble. In the years I had lived in Arizona, whenever Mother came to visit, we would always take a couple of days and visit Las Vegas. At the clinic, Mother asked Sharon and Bruce if it would be all right if we flew to Reno for the weekend and played the slot machines. They not only approved, they thought it was an excellent idea. They wanted me to start taking short trips away from the hospital. Mother was delighted, and I was happier for her than for myself. She hadn't had a break from sickness and death for months. A few days of just having a good time would do as much for her as for me.

We left the following Saturday morning. When we climbed into a cab at the Reno airport, the driver turned to look at me.

"Are you Mary?" he asked.

"Yeah," I answered.

"Well, you're lookin' good. Happy to have you in my cab." The driver had a million questions. How was I feeling? When was I released from the hospital? I smiled at Mother. At that moment, I realized that I'd have to answer such questions for the rest of my life. I didn't mind; the cab driver was cheerful and I could see his concern was genuine.

We checked into a hotel and walked down the street to a casino where Mother immediately began playing the dollar slot machines. On one of her first pulls, she hit a jackpot and let out a squeal of joy. I was happy for her. I played too, more slowly than Mother. It was all I could do to pull the handle. We were lucky, one or the other of us seemed to hit something on nearly every try. In a few minutes we had collected more than $200.

I sat back on a stool and looked around me at the people gambling. The casino was doing a nice business but was not overly crowded. Suddenly I grew afraid. It wasn't just fear, it was something more, something I couldn't describe. I wasn't afraid of the people, my surroundings, or anything I could name. If I had known the cause, maybe I could have handled it. I went into a blind panic, panic without reason, just raw fear.

I didn't want Mother to know what was happening to me. She was having such a great time shoving dollars into the machine, waiting as it clicked, and laughing as the coins she won clinked into the holder. I had to get out of there. I knew I'd break if I didn't. My panic was racing out of control. I managed to put on a poker face and told Mother, "I'm going back to the hotel."

"Are you all right?" Mother asked, pulling the handle once more. "Do you want me to come with you?"

"No, I'm okay. You stay and play," I answered. I left as quickly as I could, fighting an impulse to run from the room that now seemed so crowded and noisy. When I reached my hotel room, I locked the door and sat down on the bed. I was terrified, panic-stricken beyond anything I had ever known. I felt no pain. There was no physical sign that anything was wrong. I tried to think, but the more I thought, the more frightened I became. I called the hotel front desk and asked to have a doctor sent to my room. A short time later a medical technician came and checked me over. She took my blood pressure, which read normal. There was no sign that anything was wrong.

The technician left. Although I had been told that everything was all right, I wasn't comforted in the least. I called again and ordered coffee. While I waited, I thought to myself, "This is silly, Mary." Then it hit me: I was afraid only because I was so far from Stanford. Bruce wasn't within call.

The realization that my fears were foolish brought me no comfort at all. I was still just as terrified. The coffee came and I drank a cup, while staring out the window. Across the street I could see a row of pawnshops, their windows barred. I hated that sight. I wanted to see something I could relate to, something to cheer me.

Mother returned. She knew immediately that something was wrong.

"I'm sure scared," was the only explanation I could give.

"Maybe you're tired," Mother suggested. "Take a nap. When you wake up you'll feel better." Taking her own advice, Mother lay down on one bed and I lay on the other.

I never felt more alone in my life. I was isolated in a world no one else understood. Terror overcame me, crowding all rational thoughts out of my mind. I had no previous experience that would help me understand my reaction. I had been afraid before, but I could always identify the cause. This nameless horror nearly paralyzed me. Sleep was out of the question.

Mother woke up and we went down to dinner. My fear had not lessened. If anything it was worse. I found it difficult even to talk to her. After dinner, I couldn't wait to get back to our room; it seemed a little safer there, away from the crowds of people. I persuaded Mother to return to the casino. I felt guilty; I was ruining her fun without good reason.

When I returned to my room I called the front desk again and asked to have someone sent to my room to check my blood pressure. The technician came. My blood pressure was fine. I realized what I really wanted was to be near someone in a medical uniform.

I lay awake all night. It seemed an eternity passed before the gray of dawn appeared and brightened into day. I called Dr. Sharon Hunt at Stanford as early as I could. Hearing Sharon's voice was only vaguely reassuring. I didn't want to hear her, I wanted her there. I tried to explain my panic.

"Mary, you're all right or we wouldn't have let you go," Sharon said. "Why don't you go out? Have breakfast, play some machines, walk around, do something to take your mind off your fear." Sharon didn't suggest I return to Stanford. I knew she wanted me to face my fears, not to flee from my situation. She was right, but fleeing was the only thing I wanted to do.

I tried one more time. I accompanied Mother to the casino to try to gamble for a while. I simply couldn't cope. My mind wouldn't stay on what I was doing. I wanted to run back to Stanford. I hated the noise and confusion of the crowded casinos. I hated the barred pawnshops across the street from my hotel. I hated the town. I vowed to go back to the hotel, pack my bags, and never return to Reno again.

The moment we returned to Palo Alto I called the hospital and managed to get Bruce Reitz. Apparently he had talked to Sharon. I could hear the disappointment in his voice when he heard I was home. He was as gentle with me as ever. He listened to my problems and tried to reassure me. I felt a little comforted when Bruce promised to see what he could do.

I called Karl. It was the middle of the day and he was at work, but I called him anyway. I hate to call Karl when he's working. I've never thought it proper for a wife to call her husband at work. What can he do anyway, except worry, when he's nowhere near the problem? Only once in our marriage had I called Karl at work, when the boys ate a whole bottle of vitamins. Today, I made that once into twice. I wanted him to reassure me, somehow, from 800 miles away, to make me believe that everything was all right. Karl was confused, I could tell from the sound of his voice. I guess I couldn't blame him. If I didn't understand what was happening to me, how could he? We talked for a long time. When we hung up, I didn't feel any better.

After I talked to Karl, he called Bruce Reitz. To this day I don't know what they said, but later that afternoon Bruce called me; I was to check into the Hoover Pavilion at Stanford the next day.

I was in Hoover more than three weeks. While there, I met Dr. Larry Koran, a psychiatrist, who began to treat me for anxiety. Anxiety is what he called my state; to me it was fear. After a few days I was at least able to sleep again.

There I was. I had survived the surgery and physically I was recovering. I knew, after all that had been done to me, that I could still die. For the first time since my transplant, I really thought about death. I had come to grips with death when I was ill, but now I had been given a reprieve and I had to come to terms with it again. In retrospect, it occurred to me that the fear episode was triggered by my trip to Reno, by having to confront its huge lively crowds. Until the trip, I had been in my little cocoon, my little apartment, with just Mother around me.

Dr. Koran, who probably knows more about transplant

psychiatry than anyone else in the world, helped me a great deal. He gave me a foundation for dealing with my problems when I left the hospital. He taught me to analyze my fear objectively; to distinguish between a life-threatening situation and just plain fear. It wasn't easy because the fear never had a rational basis, but slowly I struggled through the problem.

Larry Koran and I talked about my childhood, my early religious training, and my "fall" from the church. I told him that although I did not believe in the dogma and ritual of the Roman Catholic church, or of any other organized religion, I did recognize the existence of a Supreme Being. More than once, I asked Larry, "If I believe in God, why am I having such a hard time dealing with death? Or is it that I really do not believe?"

Deep down, I still was bothered by the question of why I had lived when so many others who deserved life had died. I finally settled on a belief that comforted me: there was a Supreme Being, but no heaven or hell, other than the one we make for ourselves during our lives; there is no guaranteed path to the continuation of life.

I was also bothered by all the attention I received and the expressions of admiration from total strangers. I felt strongly that I didn't deserve it. It wasn't modesty; it was a really troubling concern. Everybody kept asking how I could be so brave. I felt like a hypocrite. I wasn't brave. I had done what almost anyone else would have done: I was dying; I had a chance to live; I took it. That wasn't bravery—I simply didn't want to die.

Dr. Koran disagreed with me. He argued that I had a right to live and that without my ability to fight, the greatest doctors in the world could not have saved me. He said I had fought for the chance to live, and after the operation, I had to find the courage and the will to stay alive. It was hard at first, but when I did accept those ideas, I started to feel better about myself.

When I was released from the hospital, I made a habit

of taking short drives. Larry Koran urged me to go a little farther each day, even if only a block. Finally, one day, Mother and I took a trip on the freeway past San Jose.

Mother couldn't drive, and driving was a problem for me. I didn't want to travel too far and I didn't like the heavy traffic. Mother kept encouraging me to go a little farther. It was hard for her, watching me struggle, hard to urge me to go farther than I wanted to, but she did it because she knew I needed to.

I talked to Karl frequently by phone. I was homesick for my family and Karl knew how important the calls were to me. He never mentioned the $400 phone bills, and for some reason, it didn't occur to me to ask how we were doing financially. I knew my medical expenses were covered by insurance, and I guess that's as far as I wanted to think about it. Karl never brought up the subject of our finances; he felt I had enough to worry about. I suppose he was right; I don't know what I could have done had he shared the problems with me. Karl had put some new household rules into effect. First, snacks were eliminated. Karl got a good deal on some tuna fish and made tuna casserole so often the boys haven't eaten it once since I returned.

He managed to cut the food bill to half of what it normally ran. I later found out that, while my men were managing to save money on the grocery bill, they were doing a good job of caring for the house. It stayed clean, except for the boys' rooms, which still would make a pigsty seem hygienic.

Those days were harder on Karl than he ever let on. He worked all day, then came home and cooked for the boys. Chris and Luke helped. They did most of the housework and seldom complained about their drastically reduced allowances, the only sign they saw of the constant financial problems that plagued Karl and which he wouldn't share with anyone. More troubling by far were their constant nagging fears about me, never really knowing how I was doing. The boys were teenagers, struggling to find themselves, trying to grow up. Not only was I not there with them, but hanging over them was the knowledge that I might die. They and Karl wanted to shield me from the problems they were having. Growing up without your mother there is hard enough without feeling you have to protect her too. They all lived on an emotional roller coaster, alternating between hope and fear. When I first became ill, they hoped a medication could help me; it didn't. When I went to Houston they hoped something could be done for me, but I returned to tell them I was dying. When I was accepted as a transplant candidate hope was born again. Then months went by without approval for the cyclosporine. I'll never know what it cost Karl to sit there holding my hand when I blacked out, never knowing whether I would live for the next five minutes. Hope returned when I had my transplant, but fear was never far away. It's hard to live for month after month on hope and fear and I think their emotions were often more stretched than the family purse. At times they all became very discouraged. Months later Karl told me that he had often asked himself where it would all end.

Now I feel terrifically selfish knowing what they all went through for me, particularly Karl. Sometimes Karl would start to feel sorry for himself because no one seemed to appreciate what he was going through, even though he wanted it that way. Remarkably, his work performance did not suffer. One of Karl's characteristics has always been the ability to separate his work from his personal life. Surprisingly, he continued to be able to do this.

At work, he faced problems that were soluble. He was working on an error correction system for satellite data transmission. The project required much intellectual activity and a creative approach. It was wonderful therapy for Karl. For a time he could escape from the tunnel that seemed to have neither light nor end.

Summer was passing. In June, Bruce Reitz had told me

I could go home the first of September, if my medical condition permitted. Wonderfully, my medical problems were few. High blood pressure presented a minor problem, but otherwise my progress was excellent. The doctors told Karl they felt the familiar surroundings of home would help combat my anxiety as much as anything. I knew they were right. I wanted to go home. Oh, did I want to go home.

In my phone calls to Karl, coming home was what I usually talked about, that and my fear episodes. He found it hard to be reassuring. He couldn't tell me, "Now, now, you're really okay." He knew I wouldn't buy such a line because I was not okay. He had to be realistic with me, although I think he wished simply to be comforting. Whatever he did, it worked. I always felt better after I talked with him, but I was still homesick.

Near the end of August I found a beautiful off-white suit with a blue blouse that I fell in love with. I wanted to look especially nice for my homecoming. Nearly everyone had thought, when I left Phoenix, that I'd never return. I was coming home and I wanted to do it in style. I called Karl. I wanted to tell him, I think, that I wanted my homecoming to be special, something neither of us would forget. And I guess I was trying to tell him I wanted to look pretty for him again. I was still a woman. But there was a bit of a pragmatist left, too, I suppose. I was vaguely aware of our money problems. I wouldn't find out for a while just how bad they were, but I knew we couldn't be doing too well. It had never happened to me before, but I felt suddenly a little guilty about wanting something as silly as a new blouse after everything Karl and everyone else had done for me during the last months. The phone was answered on the second ring.

"Karl, honey," I began. He probably knew I wanted something from my opening. "I've found a gorgeous suit and blouse I'd like to wear home. It's awfully expensive. Can we afford it?"

His heart probably sank at my words, but you'd never know it from his voice. He immediately answered, "Sure, honey. You go out and get it."

Karl had also sent airline tickets for Mother and me. They were first-class tickets. I had never flown first class in my life and I was thrilled. I called him.

"Why did you do that?"

His answer was simple. "You deserve it. Hell, everyone should go first class once in their life, and if you haven't earned the privilege, no one ever will."

I felt good.

September first came . . . John and Cheryl Hanron were coming over to take Mother and me to the airport. I dressed slowly, putting on my new suit for the first time. I was happy to be going home, but my joy was tinged with sadness. I had made many friends in Palo Alto, not just the doctors and nurses, but my neighbors and some of my fellow transplant patients. I thought of them as I dressed. They were a wonderful, courageous group of people.

Gil Macy, a heart transplant from New York City, was one of my favorites. His transplant had taken place before cyclosporin came along. The antirejection drugs had made his bones brittle, and he had broken nearly every bone in his body at one time or another. He had the puffed-up moon face characteristic of those who take steroids.

Gil visited me frequently, and during my hospital stay, his wife Estelle stopped in every day to visit my mother and take her to lunch or out for a break. Seeing Gil's struggles without the cyclosporin, I realized just how crucial a role the drug played, and how lucky I was to have benefited from it. Gil was the first patient who was changed from other drugs over to the cyclosporin. The doctors didn't really know how the changeover would affect him, but I guess they had little choice. His bones were breaking from the weight of his body. It worked wonderfully. The last time I saw him, I didn't even recognize him. He had straightened up and his face, no longer puffed up, had changed drastically. He looked terrific.

I finally finished dressing, and John and Cheryl came. We were all packed. I took a last look around the apartment, partly to be sure we hadn't forgotten anything, but mostly because I had grown to love our little place in Palo Alto. I had arrived seven months earlier with only a few weeks to live, and now I was going home. I didn't know what lay ahead. I only knew that whatever it was, I was alive to face it.

SIXTEEN

I WAS GOING HOME! AS I WALKED OUT OF THE APARTMENT building the same thought kept running through my head: I was going home. No more hospital; no more doctors; no more nurses; I loved them all, but I wanted to go home. I wanted my family around me in surroundings I could call my own. Karl and I could be together as often as we wanted. I'd have my children again, to love and to hold. They'd drive me nuts at times, I knew that, but I wanted to be with them anyway. To see them grow was one of the reasons I had fought to stay alive.

Realistically, I knew that I'd still be under a doctor's care, that I'd never again go long without medical supervision. Also, in the back of my mind the fear of leaving Stanford still gnawed away. This morning, though, I didn't care.

I felt good. I weighed ninety-four pounds, only a few pounds under my normal body weight, and although I was still weak, I could get around easily enough. John and Cheryl, ever faithful, arrived early to take Mother and me to the airport. They didn't want me to worry about being late. We needed to be early. The hospital public relations staff had warned us the media would show up. The warning—if it could have prepared us—was insufficient. The media ambushed us at the curb. Again, I was astonished at all the furor over me. I could not imagine why all these people would come all the way out to the airport to see me. A representative of United Airlines was there to rescue us from the crowd, and we were ushered to a large VIP room.

I was excited, but not particularly nervous in anticipation of meeting the press. I liked them and I thought they liked me. Oddly enough, I was far more comfortable answering their questions than I was meeting people on the street who wanted to talk to me. I was not afraid I would get a question I couldn't answer.

It was curious how the media acted during that news conference. It was not the traditional mob scene of shouting reporters I had seen on television. The reporters seemed strangely courteous, not only with me, but with each other, and they asked their questions one at a time. Later, Max Jennings, my *Mesa Tribune* editor, marveled at this. "Those don't sound like the guys I know," he said.

The only untoward incident I saw at the San Francisco news conference was a brief argument between two still photographers. One of them stepped in front of the other and they exchanged words. Except for that, every one of those people was courteous and gentle during the forty-minute interview.

As we headed through the airport on the way to the plane, Karl's favorite picture of me, of all the news photographs, was taken. I was riding in a wheelchair to the plane, because it was so far, when we ran into one of my intensive-care nurses. She was astonished to see me.

"Mary!" she yelled in greeting and came running over to me.

I threw up my hands, instantly on the defensive. I remembered how hard she had worked to get me out of a wheelchair and walking only a short time before.

"I'm only in the wheelchair because I have so far to

walk," I said. I smiled at her. I was just as proud as punch to see her there. It was a victory for both of us.

She hugged and kissed me. "Look, I could use a wheelchair to get around this place," she said, oblivious of the photographers gathered around. Karl's favorite photo shows me wearing a huge smile, my arms extended upward to the nurse. To him it somehow symbolizes my victory over death. It's a temporary victory, all victories over death are, but it's still a victory.

We climbed aboard the plane and settled into the unaccustomed luxury of the first-class seats. No sooner had I buckled my seat belt when what may be the strangest incident of all happened. The cockpit door opened and Jack Mathes was standing there. I don't know how, but I identified him instantly. Jack Mathes was the airline captain who sent one of my first cards after my surgery. On the lovely Irish card, he sent his best wishes from 39,000 feet. I hadn't forgotten that card, and the coincidence of his being the captain on my flight home was delightful. It was truly a coincidence; he hadn't known I'd be on the plane until he received the passenger manifest.

As he came up to me, he said, "Mary, you don't know me. You probably don't remember, but I sent you a card."

"Yes, I do," I said. "You sent me a lovely Irish card. I tried to call you several times, but I never could seem to reach you."

"Well, I'm your pilot today," he said.

I smiled. "Then I won't be nervous."

"Mary, I'm so proud to have you on my plane. You have a nice flight." He leaned over and kissed me on the cheek.

It *was* a nice flight. For the first time in years I wasn't nervous when flying. I'm a seat gripper when I fly. I always have been. This time I was relaxed, knowing Jack was at the controls. My world seemed crowded with friends.

During the flight, I was absorbed, thinking about my family. I was so anxious to see them I could hardly stand it.

I imagined the reactions of Karl and the kids on seeing me on my feet and walking, and ready to live again, after so many months of struggle. I wanted to show them how much I had improved! Most of all, I couldn't wait to be alone with them. I expected a few people to meet me, and I wanted to show the whole world that I had come home. At the same time, though, I was apprehensive. I had been away so long! How much time would it take us all to get back to normal? I longed for normalcy.

Several people on the plane recognized me and came over to talk. One woman was from Mesa. She wore that awe-struck look of someone who is meeting a celebrity. It made me uncomfortable. I'm not a celebrity. I'm just Mary. But the woman was nice.

"I'm from Mesa, and I've been reading all about you in the *Tribune,*" she said. "You look so good, and I'm so glad you're coming home. We've all been waiting for you." It was a sincere comment I would hear many, many more times. I have always been a "people" person, but I was still having trouble adjusting to the accolades of strangers. Why didn't they reserve their praises for Bruce? He had worked for years to save lives and he had saved mine.

When we landed in Phoenix, Jack Mathes brought the plane down like a powder puff. I was the last person to leave the plane. When I walked down the tunnel, the first people I saw were Karl and my two boys. We hugged briefly; our reunion would have to wait until later. Now, the waiting room at the airport was a mob scene. All the local television stations were there, together with the news reporters from the local papers, some from California and the wire services. It was a madhouse. Max Jennings was there to meet me, and to cover the story for the *Tribune.* Several members of my former staff had come to greet me. I was happy to see them, and Dean Gordon, one of my sales reps and a good friend, handed me a beautiful bouquet of red roses, a lovely welcome home.

The scene at the airport contrasted starkly to my memory of the day I had left. No one had wanted to see me off, they couldn't bear it. I had been dying, but now I was alive, happy to be able to hug and greet them all. Then I had been in a wheelchair and had to be carried on to the plane. Now I walked down to the room where I would have my second news conference of the day. I was still weak, but I walked.

The reporters' questions were growing predictable. Only one reporter asked me the question a lot of people were thinking, "Do you feel like a guinea pig?"

I can't remember how I answered that, but I'll never forget how I felt. I felt very much alive and I was filled with a grateful joy. I had my boys with me, my husband, my friends, and I was home. If it weren't for Bruce Reitz and everyone at Stanford I wouldn't have been there at that moment. If that's what being a guinea pig meant, then I was glad to be one.

The news conference over, we all piled into the car for the ride to Mesa. I was amused at Chris. Usually he was Mr. Stoic, but not today. He sat in the backseat, grinning from ear to ear. Luke had grown; he seemed all legs to me. It was great, being with my whole family, driving again down familiar streets, far away from the hospital.

"Do you want to stop at the paper for a minute?" Karl asked.

I thought about it a moment. I was tired, but I wanted to stop and say hello to Haney and Carole and many of the people at the paper. They had built a new building since I had left and I felt part of that building was mine. I'd worked to get it and I wanted to see it. When we pulled up in front of the paper, I realized I had been set up. This was going to involve more than just saying hello to a few people. Draped across the front of the building was a huge yellow banner, at least thirty feet long, with "WELCOME HOME MARY" in letters three feet high.

Haney Womack was pacing back and forth in front of the building when we pulled up. I guess we arrived before we were expected. Haney would have died before he would let me catch him on his feet and edgy. He would have preferred to be sitting in his office when I walked in so he could say something like, "It's about time you got back to work." I was moved, seeing him like that, nervous, concerned that everything was just right for my homecoming.

We parked in front of the building. I saw Chuck Wahlheim, the publisher, who looked just as nervous as Haney. They came over as I climbed out of the car and we walked through the front door and into the advertising department. I was stunned. The entire newspaper staff seemed to be waiting for me. I expected the advertising staff to be around, but I was astonished to see everyone else as well. All the editorial department people were there. People from the back shop were waiting to greet me. Even some of the pressmen were there, grins showing through the smeared ink on their faces. They stood in a ring that stretched around the back of the room, as if they were held back by an invisible rope. It was strangely quiet. I don't think anyone knew what to do or say; I know I didn't. I was touched by the love I could feel reaching across the space between us. I loved them back.

We stood there for a moment more, then Chris Fleur, a good friend and one of my former staff, came forward, put his arms around me, gave me a kiss, and said, "Welcome back, Mary." Pat McElfresh from the editorial staff came over and hugged me. Someone clapped tentatively, then everyone began clapping. The ice was broken, and people crowded around greeting me and wishing me a welcome home.

"What is everyone doing?" I yelled to make myself heard. "Why aren't you working?"

Everyone laughed. The mayor, Don Strauch, was present and gave me a certificate, declaring it Mary Gohlke Day in Mesa. I suppose it was corny, but I didn't think so.

I realized how little we know about the people around

us. Some of the people there I knew well, the ones I had worked with closely, but many who were crowded into that room I didn't know well: people with whom I hadn't had daily contact, whose faces were familiar, but whose names I could no longer remember. I saw them standing there, knowing they all had an idea of what I had gone through. They had come to show their support, to give a measure of their love. Their reaction was spontaneous. It wasn't pretentious, they really cared. They shared my joy in returning home and wanted me to know they were happy for me. I expected such empathy from my family and close friends, but from these people, some of them nearly strangers, it came as a shock. I was surprised and as deeply touched by their love as by anything else that had happened to me.

We all started back to view the new printing press, which had been installed while I was in the hospital. Inspection of a new press may seem like a silly thing to do on such an occasion, but not to a newspaperperson. Besides, I wanted to see it. Part of that press belonged to me; I had given much of my worklife to help earn the money to build it.

Chuck Wahlheim, as publisher, took the lead on the parade to the pressroom. He rushed ahead, too fast for me. Maybe he thought I'd been off training for the Olympics, instead of getting a transplant. Newspaper and TV photographers were clustered around, walking backward in front of us as we made our way. It was odd being photographed by "my" paper. I finally made it back to the press. It was monstrous, and although I was glad to see it, to tell the truth, I was happier to see the press foreman, Norm Miller. His smile alone was a warm welcome, and I could see he was proud of his new baby. I was happy for him.

I was so tired by the end of the tour that I wasn't sure I could make it to the car. Somehow I did. When we arrived home, a few neighbors were waiting to greet us. They had brought flowers and food. I thanked them, and was doubly thankful for their consideration when they quickly excused themselves and left. I was dead tired.

My first objective when I finally got into the house was to slip into a comfortable robe and take a nap. When I arose, I finally took a look around the house. It was spotless.

"You guys must really have worked hard. I'm surprised," I confessed. "This place is really clean."

Luke finally owned up. They had called Kathy Nelson, who used to come over and clean when I worked, to come and scrub the house down.

We sat down together and began to catch up on all the things that had happened while I was at Stanford. It would take a long time for me to get back into the routine of my own home, but we started right away. Bubbles, my adorable little fur ball of a dog, had been lost. Luke, in a stroke of genius, had put a note in every mailbox in the neighborhood. She had been found all right, two doors away. She's a cute dog and I love her, but I had to face facts. She was hardly a genius at finding her way home.

We were all tired so we went to bed early. To lay down in my own bed for the first time in nearly eight months was the perfect end to a perfect day. The ugly green oxygen tanks that had stood so long at the side of my bed were gone. I could go to sleep without fear of never waking. Karl put his arm around me as I went to sleep. It had been a long, hard road back to this bed and I was sure of one thing—the trip had been worth it.

SEVENTEEN

A STRANGER LIVED IN MY HOUSE. HER NAME WAS MARY Gohlke, and she didn't know this place. I don't know what I expected to find when I came home. What I wanted, I suppose, was for everything to be the same, the anchor in my storm, something like that.

It was a silly idea because nothing in my life ever would be the same. Things always change. I knew that intellectually. But still, little things hurt my feelings as I walked through the house I hadn't seen in so long. I had been looking forward to this moment for an eternity, but everywhere I looked there was a little shock. My dishes weren't in their accustomed places, and some had disappeared. The pots and pans were all mixed up. Some of the furniture had been moved. My linens were a hopeless jumble.

But these details didn't really bother me. I felt I had become the outsider in my own home, not really part of the family that lived there. Karl and the boys had adjusted to my being gone and obviously had been getting along just fine without me, or at least getting along. I should have reveled at that; instead, I was vaguely upset. I think I almost would have preferred to see a mess only I could straighten out. In short, I guess I didn't feel needed—loved, yes—but not needed as much as I would have liked.

Gradually—why it took so long, I don't know—I began to accept the hard truth a more logical person would have recognized instantly. Things could never be the same. Luke, in particular, was having a hard time understanding why he couldn't just snap his fingers and make everything like it used to be. He assumed because I was home, I was the same mom I had always been. We even had a few arguments when he wanted me to drive him some place and I couldn't because I didn't feel up to it. He believed I just didn't want to help him. He was fourteen, and I felt he could have been more understanding. If he only knew! No, no. I wouldn't ever want him to know everything that happened in that hospital, or even the things that were still happening in my mind.

I wanted so desperately to be a normal mother again, the kind who didn't have to prove anything to herself or to her family. But it wasn't easy. Even at home, I had to establish myself again. One day Luke asked me if he could go to the midnight movies, and I told him he was too young. He spun on his heel and went to the bedroom to call Karl at work. Karl's first question was, "Did you talk to your mother?" Luke told him yes, and Karl said firmly, "Well, do what she told you." That put an end to the problem. A small victory maybe, but even such a little thing made me feel better. I was so insecure! It would have been a meaningless little event in any other environment, but to me, it was an important victory in my battle for full self-worth.

Such little victories were too few to keep my spirits up, though. Mother was living with us, and she was just as protective as she had always been. When I tried to do something and struggled, she would move in and take care of it for me. There was just nothing for me to do. Mother could cook and clean everything faster and better than I could, so she did. She had no idea that I wanted to perform some tasks myself just to feel needed. It was more than that. In my mind my self-worth was based on what I was able to accomplish, and most of the time that was pitifully little.

The doctors at Stanford had hammered at me about the need to exercise when I got home. I have never been the jock type, at least not since my tomboy days in Buffalo, and I had never exercised in my life. My feelings didn't change just because I had undergone an operation. I didn't like exercise before, and I didn't like it now. But I knew the doctors were right, as usual. I had little stamina. I would be exhausted after a short trip to the grocery store or after having lunch with my friends. I knew that before I could go back to work I would have to build my strength. I started making trips to a nearby hospital to get help from the physical therapist.

Gradually, I grew stronger. After all, I had a lot of pressure and no excuses. Everyone—my doctors, the therapist, even my friends—had recommended that I swim for exercise. But we had no pool. In our part of Arizona, not to own a pool was almost the exception rather than the rule. Karl and I had planned to build one, but that was just one of the plans my illness interrupted. And a public pool was out of the question because of the danger of infection.

Max Jennings still wrote about me from time to time because the paper continued to get so many calls. If a few weeks passed without a story, the calls would start to come in again. In one piece written just before I came home, Max mentioned that I was exercising and that I wanted to swim regularly as soon as we could afford to put in a pool. It was an innocent remark on my part, just a dream Karl and I would consider seriously when we started to recover financially. I felt the whole family would enjoy it and hoped I would learn to like it as well. The casual mention of the pool in a single line in the newspaper story started phones ringing again. Before the day was out, there were offers from several companies to build a pool for the Gohlke family, including an offer from a Mormon youth group.

Karl called me in Stanford with the news. We were both stunned. Nobody had ever done anything like that for us before, and we didn't dream it could happen to us. Max called Karl the following day with still another offer.

The outpouring of kindness was having its effect. I had always been a pretty tough character when it came to sizing people up. At the same time, I was probably quicker to see the good in people than the bad, and I always assumed the best about a person until I had reason to think otherwise. But I basically believed most people were going to take care of themselves first, long before worrying about someone else. This assessment of human nature didn't turn out to be always accurate. It was a little hard to understand the incredibly kind things people were continually doing and saying at that time. One thing is for certain. It changed Karl and me forever. I think anyone who received such compassion from strangers would never be the same.

Delores and Gene Schuld, who owned a Mesa pool company, came over to explain to Karl what they wanted to do for us. It was quite simple. They would build a big, beautiful new swimming pool for $1! It was a hard moment for Karl. He was grateful. He knew it would be wonderful therapy for me. But it was a handout, and Karl Gohlke had never accepted a handout in his life. He just didn't know what to say or do.

But Luke did. He gleefully provided the dollar and the deal was struck! The Schulds told Karl they hoped to have the pool ready by the time I arrived. Because their business was so good, they were unable to keep that promise. I was glad because I got to see the pool installed after I got home. The workmen arrived a few days after my return, and they soon became my buddies. I went out every day and talked with the crew, a routine that reminded me of going into the pressroom at the newspaper. Only this time I didn't have to earn any respect. The crew all knew about me. I found out later that when they were talking to each other about jobs on their truck radios, or when they were planning their work at the office, it was always, "Well, we've got to do such and such at *Mary's pool.*" That's the way they looked at it—as something special they were doing for someone they wanted to help. Their attitude meant a lot more to me than the pool itself. It was another chapter in my new education about human nature. And I loved the lesson!

Although euphoric about getting home and resuming my life, I remained disappointed about my slow recovery. I had to start making a contribution to Karl and the boys again, and I had a job waiting. Believe me, in my head, I was more than eager to get on with the business of living, but my body just wouldn't answer my mental commands.

My main problem was nausea. I had so much trouble keeping my food down that I was left weak and without energy much of the time. I spent too much time in bed, and this compounded my problems as I tried to reestablish myself in the family routine. The kids didn't know whether to bother me with their requests or wait until they could talk to their father. It was a tough time for me because I wanted so desperately to take over my old responsibilities.

Ironically, what probably helped me during this time was the undeniable evidence someone out there *did* need me, even though I couldn't work or help around the house. I could answer the telephone, and my common sense hadn't deserted me. And by golly, I was alive, thank you! That was more than enough for many of the people who called me. Karl and I decided it wasn't necessary to change our phone number after I came back, and I started getting a few phone calls. Remarkably, I did not receive even one crazy call. Most of the callers were strangers who obviously had to screw up their nerve to talk to me. Some of them were ill themselves. Often they were calling for advice on what to do about an ill relative. I could never help with medical advice, of course. But I think some of them just wanted to hear my voice. My voice always has been relatively strong, and without exception, people would tell me, "You sound great!" Even on days when I was feeling lousy, people would still tell me this. I sensed I was a source of comfort to them, although I felt sorry for many. They thought that by talking to me some kind of magic would rub off and they would be okay.

I think I took just about every call. I knew instinctively it was good therapy; it made me quit thinking about myself, and I felt I was able to do some good for most of those reaching out to me.

Still, it was hard to talk to some people because they had no idea what I was going through, and I suppose I found it difficult to identify with their particular problems. My own illness was so rare it was hard to find anyone who had ever heard of it; it wasn't like talking to a fellow cancer patient. It was painfully easy now for me to remember how desperately I had wanted to talk to *anyone* who might understand just a little of what I was going through, especially about the times when I was afraid. I couldn't talk about this and be really honest because many of those calling me for help already were terrified either for themselves or their loved ones. Often they asked how I kept going before my surgery, and if I was ever tempted to just give up. Oh, how I understood the question! My answer always was the same; I told them I set goals for each day. The big one was to try to stay alive until I could undergo surgery. Another one was to see the kids grow up. I didn't lie to them; I didn't tell them it was a charming yellow brick road I went down. I told these faceless new friends that there were days when I felt awful and that I had to take things one step at a time. Not profound, maybe, but that's the way it was.

Well, mostly. Maybe I was a little hypocritical because I

wasn't feeling too good about myself when I was trying to help the callers. I was sitting on my tail too much. I wasn't very motivated, and I didn't like this about myself. It wasn't my style. I realized I had to grab on to the physical part of getting better—get some exercise, push myself—but I just didn't want to. Mother and I took walks, and Karl and I went to lunch a few times. I still didn't like it when people came up to me at lunch or on the street. People weren't mean or rude, but I still didn't understand why it was such a big deal to talk to me.

One day as I was buying a handbag at a department store, the very young woman behind the counter was complaining about working on such a beautiful day. As she wrote up the ticket, she saw my name. "Gosh, you're the last person I should be complaining to," she said. I smiled.

"Well, why don't you have your lunch outside today?" I suggested. "It is beautiful out there. You would enjoy that."

"You know, I will," she said. I think she probably did. I felt good about my little lecture. I was getting better at relating to people; I was preparing myself to go back to work. I had really become a recluse, and I didn't like that change. It simply had become easier to stay away from people than to learn to deal with them under my new status.

The other thing that worried me was my weight. Try as I might, I couldn't keep it up. I weighed well under ninety pounds now, and I never was excited about eating. It was a funny feeling, but after just a few bites of even my favorite foods, it would feel as if I had had a huge meal and I just couldn't continue.

I was impatient at my lack of progress, but I never forgot for a moment the enormous difference between this year and the previous one. It seemed impossible that a year ago I was dying and without hope! Death was on the back burner now, and my concerns were of another type.

Christmas descended upon the Gohlke family before

we were ready. It was a vastly happier time than the year before when the unspoken idea it could be our last together was uppermost in our minds. But this year I was a little bit blue because our family Christmas didn't resemble the one on the Hallmark Card with the family gathered 'round the fireplace. I was unreasonably disappointed simply because this Christmas wasn't *perfect.* I guess, for whatever reason, I felt I deserved a perfect Christmas.

We exchanged gifts and had a nice time, but Chris was getting ready to go on a skiing trip, our present to him, and Luke was with his friends most of the time. I don't know what I expected, but I wasn't being realistic in hoping we would all sit around and hold hands all day or whatever image I had in my mind.

As usual, Karl was incredibly thoughtful. Years ago I had lost my wedding ring. It was not covered by insurance, and we certainly couldn't afford to replace it. We had one little child and were trying to fix up our house. But this Christmas Karl replaced it in style! The ring had a ruby, flanked by two diamonds in a beautiful custom setting.

Karl's gift wasn't the only precious one. Joyce Howland, always one of my dearest friends, gave me a turquoise heart inset with an outline of lungs in gold and a diamond heart. It was a gift to be treasured, one to remind me constantly of my greatest gift of all—the additional years of life I had been given.

I had hoped that after the holidays, when things were back to normal, I would start gaining weight, but the problem was getting worse. I suffered bouts of nausea, and it was obvious to me that I needed some more help. My regular checkup at Stanford was scheduled in January, and I returned there both dreading it and hoping at the same time to find out what was wrong with me. I was almost sure it had nothing to do with my heart and lungs, but I certainly wanted that confirmed.

The familiar surroundings of the Stanford Medical Center brought home to me how many tests I would have to go through. This time I wasn't naive! I knew what to expect. They were waiting for me, and the tests began almost as soon as I walked through the door.

One of the first was to see how efficiently my heart and lungs were functioning. They inserted a shunt in my artery and put me on a treadmill at a certain speed. The shunt was a needle with a tiny valve that allowed blood samples to be taken repeatedly without reinserting the needle. I was grateful that the device spared me repeated punctures, although I hated to have it inserted. Worse, while I was on the treadmill, I had to breathe through a tube so the amount of lung capacity could be checked.

With shunt and breathing tube in place, I walked on the treadmill for a while, stopped while they drew blood, and then resumed walking. The oxygen content of my blood at various exercise levels would give a rather exact picture of just how well my transplanted organs were working. This procedure, although never painful, was damned exhausting.

The next day's event was a catheterization to double-check circulation through the heart. First they strapped me into the "canoe," which resembled a hammock. At the same time as one group was working the catheter through the artery in my leg into my heart, another doctor inserted into my jugular vein a tiny wire with a little clamp on the end to snip a piece of the transplanted heart tissue.

If all this weren't enough, someone handed me a bicycle wheel device with handles and ordered me to pump away while they were working on me from two directions. It was almost too much to bear. I turned my head to see Sharon Hunt, who rapidly was becoming one of my favorite doctors. She was intent on her work, and I felt she had forgotten me for a moment. I snapped at her. "Who invented this goddamned medieval torture device?" She barely smiled. She knew I thought it was one of the worst experiences I had ever had, and she was right!

I was conscious during the entire procedure, and it was

a miserable experience, just as bad as Chuck Walker had predicted. Chuck, who had received his heart-lung transplant after I had obtained mine, called me the day before my test to tell me what to expect. The doctors were furious when they learned about this. Chuck's call worried me so much I had trouble sleeping the night before. Unfortunately, the worry was justified.

But the good news was not long in coming. The transplanted heart was working fine, the lung capacity had increased, and in every respect, the newest parts of my body were doing just fine! There apparently was no rejection.

Next, I wanted to find out about my eating problem. The specialists decided to give me a complete gastrointestinal examination. The doctors soon found a ball of hair and undigested fiber in my stomach. They theorized that my antirejection drug, the cyclosporin, could have contributed to the problem because it promotes hair growth. The doctors were sure the ball interfered with my digestion and also contributed to my "full" feeling, which kept me from eating. But how to get rid of it was another question.

It took a week to make the decision. Surgery might have been the logical option for a normal person. But because my immune system was suppressed, any infection brought on by the surgery could be fatal. They decided to go down my esophagus with an instrument and break up the ball in my stomach.

Karl had gone home, but he flew back for this next crisis. I was prepared for major surgery and put to sleep. Unfortunately, attempts to break up the hair ball failed, and the next problem for the doctors was to decide immediately where to cut into the stomach and how much actual cutting would be necessary.

After another huddle, the doctors decided to make a small slit in my stomach and remove the ball. While they were at it, they rebuilt my pylorus, the opening from the stomach to the intestine. Any kind of surgery of this kind is dangerous because of infection: in my case, it was extremely dangerous. But it also was remarkably successful. I suffered no complications and I returned to Mesa on the following Tuesday. I felt great! I started to gain weight and get my strength back. Mentally, I was up. I was getting ready to go back to work. I was back!

EIGHTEEN

HANEY WOMACK TOLD ME HE WANTED ME TO RETURN TO work on March 9. It may have been coincidental, but I'll always wonder if my tough general manager wasn't the most sentimental person in our building. Whatever his reasoning, I was ready to return exactly one year to the day after Bruce Reitz had opened my chest to try to accomplish a feat no surgeon had ever done before. My dream of being able to return to work was one of the reasons Bruce and I had made our pact, and on the day the promise came true, I was ready. I owed no apologies to anyone. After all I had been through, I felt I had earned my second chance.

Haney and Chuck Wahlheim, now Cox Arizona president, and I agreed I would first work at our sister Cox paper in Tempe, which faced sales problems. We decided to try it for thirty days and see what happened. Even the preliminary planning was exciting for me. I was using my mind for a change instead of being preoccupied with my body.

I dressed carefully that first morning, my mind racing with plans for the day. I felt absolutely wonderful. I was strong and alert. I felt up to any challenges. I drove to

Tempe, trying to recall the names and faces of the advertising people who worked there. The first person I saw when I arrived at the *Tempe Daily News* parking lot was Buster Sumpter, a pressman I've known for years. "Hey, Mary!" he yelled at me. He came over and threw his arms around me. I was glad I ran into a familiar face first thing. It was the kind of welcome I'd hoped for.

I walked through the back of the plant, stopping to speak to people as I went. I received many curious stares, but I expected that. The day raced by. I visited with each of the salesmen and attacked the first problem I came across—the filing system. It was a mess and obviously was affecting the productivity of the entire department. After assigning a staff member to the problem, I worked through a few other matters, and the day was over before it seemed possible. I was not as tired as I had feared, and it felt good to be back!

My "celebrity" status interfered somewhat during those first days. I could tell people sometimes weren't relating to me as a boss or an advertising director, but as the person who had had "the operation." Also, quite frankly, the advertising staff wasn't used to the tempo I set. I pushed them almost from the first day, and the resentment that resulted complicated an already touchy situation. But we worked through it, and my self-confidence began to soar. I had always been good at this job, and the operation hadn't changed that.

Before my thirty-day trial period was up, I was transferred back to the *Mesa Tribune* to take over my old duties as advertising director. The transfer was another reinforcement. It wouldn't have happened if I had not been getting the job done. Too many dollars were at stake. On top of the transfer, I received another small but important little boost for my ego. One of the bright young women in our business office, Diane Davison, told me I had been selected as the Woman of the Year by the Tempe chapter of Business and Professional Women.

I was flattered, but worried slightly about the acceptance speech. I asked my "word man," Max Jennings, how to write it. His advice was instant. "Don't write any fancy speech," he said. "Just tell it like it is. You're good at that."

I did. The banquet was held at a Tempe restaurant, and many of the people in the audience, to my delight, were media buyers. I did a little selling job on them, I confess. I told them why newspaper advertising was so effective, and I answered many questions. Throughout that evening, there was not one mention of my operation, or of my "celebrity" status. That wasn't why I was there. I was there because I was a successful professional woman, and they wanted to hear me talk. The distinction meant a lot to me; for the first time in a long time, I wasn't Mary Gohlke, medical freak, but Mary Gohlke, advertising executive. That's what I wanted. Their view of me as noteworthy businesswoman meant more to me than the award. I wish I could have bottled up all the self-confidence and reinforcement I felt that night and taken it back to work with me.

My office at Mesa had been remodeled in my absence, and it was nearly twice as big. I needed the space because the job had grown more demanding while I was gone. I slipped fairly easily back into the routine I knew so well. But just as at home, things had changed. I couldn't do anything about that.

I could sense that the employees, not just in my department but everywhere in the building, were having trouble relating to me in the way they had before. Some of them would scarcely look me in the eye, and people seemed to be afraid to disagree with me. We weren't playing by the usual rules, and I didn't like the change. I didn't expect special treatment. I had a job to do, and that's all I wanted. But at the same time I recognized it was not easy just to wipe away everything that had happened to me. I only had to look in the mirror.

I was tiny. I was frail. My eyes were enormous and

liquid, and they dominated my face, which still was a little puffy from all the drugs. I was not the same person I was before the operation, as much as I wanted to be. My name continued to pop up on television and in local publications from time to time. But I was determined not to let that get in the way. I started to make sales calls, and there was a certain tension there, too. Some of the customers really wanted to ask me about my operation, but they were afraid to. I could tell that.

Gradually, the gloves came off around the office, though. The advertising department had put together a special section, and we had most of the ads ready. The section was a dandy piece of work from the ad staff and would bring in a significant amount of extra revenue. It needed only minor support from editorial to lay out the pages and put in a few stories. At least that's the way I looked at it; Max usually didn't agree the job was so easy. In this case, when I checked on the section two days before it was supposed to go to press, editorial had done nothing. I went storming into Max Jennings's office and interrupted a phone conversation.

"Why in the hell hasn't this been done?" I demanded. "Editorial hasn't even started."

Max yelled across the city room to his managing editor, Peter Friedrich, and he and Friedrich promptly got into an argument. When the smoke cleared, I had the promise that editorial would take care of my section that day. One for the little lady!

After that incident my relationship with Max went right back to normal. Others didn't understand this. One day I was standing in a narrow hall talking to someone when Max came by. "Get your little butt out of the way," he demanded without a trace of humor in his voice. I meekly complied, and he winked at me as he passed. The person I was talking with was outraged. She had no idea he was just being friendly.

About this time Max and I decided to write a book together. I had a story to tell, and he knew me about as well as anyone outside my family and close friends, and besides, he had written more about me than anyone else. He had written numerous columns and stories, and his article in *Ladies Home Journal,* which appeared the month after I came home, drew mail from everywhere. Max told me several times I was the most honest person he had ever interviewed.

We met at 7 A.M. every Thursday at the office, and Max would interview me for an hour. During one interview while I described having to tell the kids I was dying, Max started to cry. His eyes got all wet, and he took out a handkerchief and wiped his eyes. Then I started to cry, watching him, and someone came into Max's office to ask him a question. There we sat, crying our eyes out. We must have made quite a sight! It was rather embarrassing, but we didn't care. It was a special moment we had shared. I often found it painful to work through these interviews, remembering the darkest days. But our conversations were a catharsis, too. I think they helped me find a perspective I hadn't had before.

Quickly, Max and I learned to work together very well during our interviews, and we determined that my story would be as honest and straightforward as we could possibly make it. This project gave a second dimension to my life. I felt I had something to say about transplants, and I hoped I would get the forum to do so. I hoped the truth of what I had gone through would be of some help. I think Max felt the same way.

Things were going reasonably well with the newspaper. We were on our budget as far as advertising sales were concerned. But there were days when I had to go home early. I was doing okay in the head, but some days my body would just poop out. I would run out of energy early in the afternoon, and there was nothing I could do. I still felt I was making a contribution. I knew I was. It was my job to bring in the budgeted revenue, and I was doing that.

One October morning, I was summoned to an unexpected meeting in the publisher's office. I'd known Chuck Wahlheim a long time, and one glance at his expression told me this was going to be bad. But I still didn't know what to expect.

"Mary, we're going to move you up to major accounts," he said, looking me in the eye. The statement took me by surprise because no one had said anything to me about being unhappy with my work.

"Is this a lateral arabesque?" I asked. My voice was calm, but I was churning inside.

"Yes." Chuck was impassive.

I was confused. I knew we needed to make some changes in that department. But I had no idea why I was being replaced. In advertising, performance is measured by numbers, and my numbers were good.

"We have four people up there in major accounts and nothing is happening," Charlie said. "We want you to turn them around and start making a profit."

Then he added the clincher I've never forgotten. "Mary, I want to exploit you." Those words rang in my ears. Charlie didn't seem to notice their effect on me. He explained he wanted to take advantage of the fact that I was a "name"—a fact which could be used to open the doors of a lot of advertisers. I was outraged, particularly at his use of the word *exploit.* What did he think I was! Charlie later explained to Max that what he meant was that I could get in to see major advertisers because of my former position as advertising director and because I was well known, when other salesmen could not. He said that was what he meant by *exploit.*

The thing that really burned me was the way in which I was demoted, if that's what it was. I have always dealt with everyone directly, and I think people who know me understand I like to be dealt with in a straightforward fashion. No one had expressed any displeasure with my performance since I came back, and I was perfectly willing to discuss my shortcomings, whatever they were.

I was damned mad that my good friend Chuck, my boss of many years who had supported me through my ordeal, had handled me this way. My pride was hurt. The nuns from my school days were right. I probably did have too much pride for my own good.

In fairness to Chuck, he had no frame of reference. I've since discovered that most people find it almost impossible to deal with a transplant; it's such a dramatic event, and they can relate only to that, not the person. I was reminded of what several other transplant recipients had told me. They weren't really given a chance to return to work. They were offered half pay or a demotion without being given a chance to show what they could do before that decision was made. Of course, some transplant recipients can't return to their previous jobs, but some of them can. I know one woman who works sixty hours a week. I guess I'm saying Chuck couldn't relate to me.

The timing couldn't have been worse. I had planned to tell Chuck and Haney later in the day that I would have to go into the hospital to be treated for a viral infection I couldn't seem to whip. The local doctors had decided I would have to be hospitalized and medicated in a controlled environment. I told Chuck and Haney I would take over my new duties in a few days when I got out of the hospital. That was a promise I couldn't keep.

I had been to the valley, and I had been back to the mountain when I came back to work, and now I was going down again. I didn't dream how bad it would be. My local doctors told me after I had been in the hospital a few days in Scottsdale that they wanted me to quit work and rest for a few months to regain my strength. They were convinced—I wasn't—that my work schedule had contributed to my run-down condition. But for whatever reason, I had to admit I had grown weaker. Maybe it was the damned viral infection; maybe it was something else, but I knew my will and determination to work could no longer triumph over my physical condition. It even occurred to me that my disappointment at my demotion—that's what I considered it—played a role in slowing my recovery. Whatever the reasons, I was sliding, and I had to concentrate on stopping it.

I made a call to Haney to tell him I would have to take a few months off. It was a terribly painful thing to do. I was out of the hospital in a few days, but this time I had no job to go back to. The only thing I had to face was sitting at home with nothing to do. I started feeling a little better, but at the same time I lost my enthusiasm for doing much of anything. I didn't particularly enjoy shopping or little excursions. I didn't even read as much, although reading had always been my passion. I don't know why I was so lethargic; I wasn't pleased with myself, and I could tell Karl was upset. He didn't like seeing me in such a condition, but he couldn't seem to reach me or interest me in anything.

Mother still lived with us, and she did much of the work around the house. The boys were busy with their own lives. I was bored, but I was enjoying the work on the book. Max came over regularly, and we recorded long interviews. He was constantly amazed by my memory. And we were making progress. That was encouraging to me.

In June, Max invited me to a dinner party at his house with Carole Doyle, my former secretary, and her husband, Bill, a physicist and an interesting conversationalist. After dinner, we returned to the living room and Max handed me a little gift-wrapped jewelry case that had been on his mantle all evening. I had noticed it but paid no attention.

I opened it to find eighteen crisp new hundred dollar bills! Max and I had agreed to split everything we made from anything he wrote about me, and more than a year before we had sold a story to a German news magazine.

The only problem after that was getting paid. With Carole's help, Max had been crusading for a year to get our money. His efforts finally paid off, and the dinner party present was his way of telling me. I felt good because I was earning money again. That was my idea of how to end a party!

As far as throwing a party myself, it was out of the question. Karl had always liked to entertain, as I knew, but I just wasn't up to it. I can't explain why. Even Luke picked up on my resistance. Luke, Karl, and I were driving down the street one day, and Luke said out of the clear, "Mother, why don't you and Dad go out and party like my friends' parents do?" Go out and have a good time was what he was trying to say. You would feel better and I would feel better. Luke was right; I needed to let my hair down a bit, but I just couldn't.

When doctors at the University of Utah decided to put an artificial heart into Barney Clark, I found myself again in the news. I gave several interviews in reaction to the Barney Clark story. In many ways, I felt I could identify with him because he was doing exactly the same thing I was: he was trying to live the best way he knew how, and in the process he was making a contribution to mankind.

I still think Barney Clark agreed to the implant of the artificial heart, which required him to be connected permanently to a bulky life-support system, because he didn't want to die. He had a choice of dying or going for the long shot. I understood what he was doing, and I applauded him for that, and the doctors for trying.

I also have to admit my choice was a lot easier than Barney Clark's. He knew he would never enjoy anything like a normal life after his operation. My case was different. I think I can say—I certainly don't know—that I would turn down an operation for an artificial heart. But I can't be sure. If I were confronted with certain death, I still might be willing to live any way I could.

In June 1983, I went back to Stanford for another

routine checkup and was found to be in good condition. My heart and lungs continued to perform perfectly, but my weight had dropped to an alarming seventy-six pounds. I was lectured on my eating habits and sent home. I failed to improve, and in July I found myself at Stanford again. This time they concentrated not on my body but on my mind. Dr. Larry Koran spent a lot of time with me, and it was obvious to us all that my weight problem was more mental than physical.

I now think they correctly diagnosed the problem. I was depressed about having to leave work. I was terribly unmotivated. And all of this was contributing to my lack of appetite. I gained seven pounds in just a few days while I was at Stanford, and on my frame, that was a lot. I came back home in a much better mental condition. I was more forward-looking and more eager to get on with life. Yet I also had to admit to myself I still had some self-doubt. I was not working. I was not really achieving much of anything except perhaps the small contributions I was making to family life.

I still received telephone calls and mail, mostly from ill people who somehow thought I could help them. I tried to talk to all of them as honestly as I could, and I still believe I helped some of those people. But I didn't do it by giving them false hope. I never did that.

My life since the transplant operation hasn't been different in some respects from the life of any other person. There are good days and bad ones. There are highs and lows. There are joys and sorrows. Life extracts a certain price. But I can say that I'm truly happy. Although I don't keep up the pace I once did, I have the energy to do many of the things I enjoy: driving, cooking, shopping, entertaining friends, caring for my family. One thing is for certain: if Bruce Reitz came to me and said, "Mary, something has gone wrong and we're going to have to do another double transplant," I'd agree to it in a second. That's because the way I know it now, living is better than dying. A lot better.

I don't know any more than anyone else why I became the first person who was allowed to live when both heart and lungs failed. I do think there are reasons. One of them, I believe, is that I was intended to share my experience with others, as maudlin as that sounds. I feel there are many, many questions I had to answer for all the terminally ill persons who wrote and called me.

I was the only one who could share their loneliness and heartache. When I was dying, I discovered what it was really like to be alone, and I could talk to those who reached out to me as no one else could. I think I've helped a lot of people. I don't know for sure, but I think I've given hope to a few—maybe that's not the best word. Maybe it's determination. I've told lots of people you have to fight, you can't give up. I think coming from me, that doesn't ring hollowly as it might coming from someone else.

Maybe I was allowed to live because of a contribution I could make to medical science. Experts in medical science know more now because of my experience. And some day we will have a National Donor Day in this country to focus attention on the need for more donors. There is an appalling national ignorance about donors. And there are legal problems at every turn. Every day lives are being lost, not because of a lack of donors, but because of the incredible legal maneuvering that has to take place before a doctor or a hospital is willing to perform a transplant. While all the papers are being filled out and signed, people are dying needlessly. Something can be done, and it must. I have seen estimates that if we had all the legal roadblocks out of the way, and if we had a good system of donor banks and national coordination, 2,000 more successful transplants could be performed each year. A better way to look at it is that we could save 2,000 lives.

To those who say transplants aren't worth the costs, I ask them what a life is worth. And transplants, even today, are cost-effective. A liver transplant is cheaper in the long run than prolonged dialysis. And we have only begun.

To Ofelia Jones, who somehow managed to think of

others in her time of grief, I owe my life. It was she who realized that by my living, her son's death would not be in vain. It took great courage for her to make her son's heart and lungs available to me, and great vision. What she did makes her, in my mind, a great person. I've never thanked her publicly before, although I've wanted to do so many times. Frankly, the doctors didn't think it would be the best thing for us to become too close, because of the psychological effects on a donor's family of knowing the identity of the recipient. But now I can express my profound gratitude and that of my family.

I honestly can say, too, that I know I would do the same thing in a moment if something happened to Karl or Chris or Luke; no one would have to ask me if their organs could be donated. I'd make the arrangements myself immediately. That's because I know how important it is. Desperate people are out there waiting, and dying, mostly because the public doesn't understand about donations. If I succeed in getting only this message across to as many people as possible, the extra years of life I have been given will be well served.

I would never condemn any person who said no to a donor request. I don't think anyone can judge. But I just want to make sure that everyone who may be able to say yes to an organ donation is at least *asked.*

I think I can say these words, too, for Bruce Reitz and all of those who have dedicated their lives to this frontier of medical science: certainly the transplant specialists are carrying out medical research. But they're also trying as much as anyone else in medical science to save lives, too.

I knew from that first electrifying moment we met that Bruce Reitz would give me life again. I knew it in my gut, and I knew it intellectually. I knew I was the first one he was going to save. I am grateful to be the one chosen by this enormous talent, but I think we both deserve a little credit, and I'm not bashful about saying so. We were stubborn; we both had courage, perhaps Bruce the greater of the two, for he was risking in a sense his own reputation. He did not know he could pull it off. He did not know what the reaction of the world would be. I, on the other hand, risked nothing. The only thing I offered Bruce was my conviction that I had a right to live, at any cost. I was not naive about what I was asking from Karl, the boys, and my mother. I was asked bluntly by Max Jennings once if I felt I had a right to demand so much of my family. He seemed a little embarrassed about asking me, but it was a question that needed answering. I suppose I could say it was incredibly selfish to ask so much. First, I was trying to survive, any way I could. I was fighting! But at the same time, I felt justified in asking for their sacrifice because I knew I had much to give if allowed the time. I think I have lived up to that. I have watched the boys grow into men, and I like to think I helped them along the way.

But after this is said, I don't know how my family stayed by me. It was a remarkable contribution from all of them—physical, emotional, financial. The sacrifice they made involves many more dimensions than this. I think the transplant team at Stanford expected my family to be heroic. And no one was disappointed. Bruce knew that without my family I wouldn't make it. He was right, as he was on so many things.

But I may be the only one who knows the full contribution of the nurses at the Stanford Medical Center. Those nurses gave me *loving* care. I would find out during my recovery that the transplant nurses have to be rotated into other areas from time to time because they become victims of emotional burnout. They are encouraged to identify with their patients, maybe even to love them if they can, and in a transplant ward, this kind of devotion has its price. But my nurses were willing to pay it, and they take a place on an equal pedestal with Bruce Reitz in the psychological support they gave me. I can't really explain it. But I *know* without the emotional investment, I would have perished.

I know this as most people will never know it. They never provided unreasonable hope. They just provided a reason to go on each day, in practical terms I couldn't deny. I've many times quoted a line from *Auntie Mame* that goes something like: "Life is a banquet, and most poor suckers are starving to death."

That's because I know, now—not before—about life. I was driving down the street the other day, the route I have taken a thousand times before, when I passed those brilliantly blooming lilac bushes. Something snapped in my mind. They were the same ones I had passed a thousand times before. But I suddenly remembered seeing them on a particular morning, the day of the floods, when a doctor I scarcely knew told me I was going to die.

Ah hah! He had been wonderfully, gloriously, stupendously wrong! I slammed on my brakes and stopped in the middle of the street. I sat there, just drinking up the beauty. A car stopped behind me, honking wildly. Other cars whizzed by, their drivers staring. I was grinning. Just grinning so big I thought my face was going to pop.

I'm alive. No, I'm more than alive. I'm living!